LIVING

The Chiropractic Way

To Brooke

The Complete Lifetime Wellness Guide

Brad Burke, D.C.

The author, editors, and publisher are not responsible for errors or omissions or for consequences from application of the book, and make no warranty, expressed or implied, in regard to the contents of the book. Any practice described in this book should be applied by the reader in accordance with professional standards of care used in regard to the unique circumstances that may apply in each situation. The reader is advised to always check product information and package inserts for changes and new information regarding dose and contraindications before administering any product.

First published by Dog Ear Publishing
4010 W. 86th Street, Ste H
Indianapolis, IN 46268
www.dogearpublishing.net

ISBN: 1-59858-085-X

This book is printed on acid-free paper.

Printed in the United States of America

"The best new book out on wellness habits and philosophy is Living The Chiropractic Way by Dr. Brad Burke. He has a superb grasp on the practical side of wellness, yet entices the reader to think outside the norm and stretch to consider the possibilities. By thoroughly addressing the concerns of the wellness consumer, including inside information on fitness and nutrition, cutting edge psychology, and the proper applications of modern chiropractic care, he paints a picture of healthy lifestyles that is attainable by anyone willing to invest the time and energy. This is a gem, and no wellness library is complete without it."

—Dennis Perman, D.C.

"When you were born,
you cried and the world rejoiced.

Live your life so that when you die,
the world cries and you rejoice."

Cherokee saying

ABOUT THIS BOOK

Your chiropractor is your Wellness expert. The fact they provided you this book speaks volumes about their commitment to your health and Wellness. They offer a wealth of expertise that can help you improve the quality of your life in ways you may not yet know. Take advantage of their clinical expertise as well as their role as your Wellness coach.

This book is designed to *expand*, not replace, your chiropractor's role in your overall Wellness. It serves this purpose in three ways.

1. By providing a wealth of information in all areas of health and Wellness. This gives your chiropractor the opportunity to help you use the tools in your life, to add further distinctions, and to expand the topics into more detailed recommendations.

2. By giving you access to Wellness information 24/7. You can learn and use the information at your own pace and in the comfort of your own home.

3. By assisting your chiropractor in determining your primary areas of need.

This book contains a powerful message and valuable tools. What you learn from that message and gain from the tools depends upon your commitment to yourself, your family, and your life.

This is a *workbook*. There are many exercises for you to do along with the information provided. The book itself provides a wealth of knowledge. However, taking an active role by completing the exercises will do far more than simply reading. Your active involvement will turn this knowledge into practice. By allowing your chiropractor to take an active role in your Wellness, you will have the ability to create the life of your dreams.

How you travel through the book is up to you. Some people like to read through everything, then go back to focus on individual chapters. Others may wish to focus on the individual chapters and exercises that best fit their current needs. The Wellness Profile (Chapter 4) will help you in this regard. Whatever approach you take, use this book to its full advantage. Read other recommended books. Follow recommendations provided by your chiropractor. Then watch your life expand in many dimensions.

The average American reads less than one book per year. The majority of times people begin a book, they fail to read past the first chapter. Far more people take Prozac, Zoloft, or other psychotropic medications than have ever read a personal development book, listened to an inspiring CD, or attended a life management seminar. Children receive thousands of hours of "education", but are rarely if ever taught how to set goals, discover a purpose for their life, balance a checkbook, or invest money.

Most people believe that we learn the "important" stuff in school. Wrong. We learn about *academics* in school. We learn about *life* in the real world. While academics are important, what we learn about *life* and *how to live* has a far greater influence on our worldly adventure.

So the first secret of life is to ***never stop learning about yourself and the world around you; never stop creating an even better version of yourself.***

Acknowledgements

First and foremost, I would like to thank The Masters Circle for their endless dedication to excellence and their vision for the future. Without their guidance, this book would have been impossible.

We should all be grateful for D. D. Palmer, who discovered the powerful healing profession of chiropractic, his son B. J. who brought chiropractic to the masses, and to the large number of chiropractors who were willing to go to jail rather than sacrifice their chiropractic ideals. Without their efforts, you would not have the freedom to gain the awesome benefits of chiropractic today.

I acknowledge the many leaders in the field of human development, including Anthony Robbins, Dennis Perman, Deepok Chopra, Wayne Dyer, Brian Tracy and many others. Through their wisdom I have gained the ability and inspiration to create this book and live my life full out.

Finally, the chiropractor that provided this book deserves a great deal of credit. They obviously care very deeply about your health and wellness and the quality of your life.

Table Of Contents

INTRODUCTION

You are about to enter a new frontier. A place you may have visited, but likely haven't stayed for long. If you are like most, you've driven past a few times. But what you saw looked too good to be true. So you just kept on driving—back to the ordinary world. A world you are more accustomed to and more comfortable in.

What is this new frontier? This is not a place, not on any map. Rather, it is a state of being, a way of living, a way of expressing and experiencing life. It is the new frontier of *Wellness*.

Wellness isn't necessarily easy, at least not in the beginning. But it is one of the most rewarding experiences you will ever have. In fact, *all of your other experiences* will change, once you truly swim in the pool of Wellness.

Some of you will jump right in. That's great! The water is safe and warm. Others of you will dip your toes for a while before fully engaging. That's ok, too. Wellness is not black and white, all or none, yes or no. It is the sum total of all of the things you can do to create the body, mind, spirit, and life of your dreams.

The journey will be filled with highs and lows, sunshine and storms, successes and "failures". But you will be rewarded with health and abundance. So enjoy the journey. Your journey to Wellness. Your journey to all that life has to offer!

FOREWORD

This book provides an honest look at two widely differing philosophies of health and life.

Wellness is the approach to health which has been promoted by Chiropractic and other natural health disciplines for over 100 years. Wellness is holistic, meaning that it is intended to improve multiple facets of health in the whole person. Wellness is so far outside the field of Medicine, that it is not even defined in most medical dictionaries. It can best be defined as *a system of health care and lifestyle which produces a condition within the body most compatible with health and healing.* Wellness-oriented approaches work *with* natural processes.

Allopathy is an approach to health dominated by fighting diseases. It is the approach used by the medical profession (allopathic medicine). Allopathy is defined as *a system of therapeutics in which diseases are treated by producing a condition incompatible with or antagonistic to the condition to be treated.* In other words, allopathic medicine *competes against* natural processes.

This book holds few punches. Everything in the book has been properly researched and is based upon the best available scientific information. However, it is written as a guidebook, not a scientific text. This is designed to keep it reader friendly.

In the course of sharing information from the vitalistic point of view, and to point out important differences between the fields of Medicine and Chiropractic, it is necessary to include information which may be unfavorable to the medical point of view. If the medical establishment is unwilling to right its own wrongs, then the informed consumer will be required to do it for them.

There are thousands of caring, responsible M.D.s and D.O.s across America and the rest of the world. In no way do I intend to downplay their role in their patients' health. Nor do I question the caring and compassion that drove them to the health care industry. Rather, it is the all powerful, arrogant and dogmatic *Pharmaco-medical Industry* that is my intended target. I also take issue with the epidemic of irresponsibility, overuse and misuse of medications and surgeries, and the unwillingness of the medical profession to allow room for any divergent viewpoints. Finally, I am appalled by the blatant lies and misrepresentations that have been directed at Chiropractic and other non-medical approaches by a small minority of medical doctors. These doctors obviously spend little time studying the scientific literature.

If you are in the medical profession, or know someone who is, please do not take my words personally. In fact, I would hope that this book would give you pause to re-evaluate outdated medical theories, and to re-think what you recommend and say to your own patients. I also hope that you can gain a new understanding of Chiropractic and the wide-ranging benefits that non-allopathic health disciplines have provided to hundreds of millions of people worldwide.

This book offers alternatives to the medical way of life. It does not undermine the value of allopathic medicine in areas where Medicine is necessary or beneficial. As a chiropractor, I immediately refer patients to a medical doctor if I have any indication they may have a medical crisis. I would hope that more medical doctors would refer patients to a chiropractor if they have any indication of vertebral subluxation.

Brad Burke, D.C.

PART 1

DEFINING WELLNESS

Chapter 1

The Wellness Revolution

"The sickness business is *reactive*. Despite its enormous size, people become customers only when they are stricken by and react to a specific condition or ailment. No one really wants to be a customer."

"The Wellness business is *proactive*. People *voluntarily* become customers—to feel healthier, to reduce the effects of aging, and to avoid becoming customers of the sickness business. Everyone wants to be a customer of this earlier-stage approach to health."

Paul Zane Pilzer, *The Wellness Revolution**

What a difference a decade can make. Just ten years ago, if you said *Wellness*, people would look at you like you had green skin and an antenna protruding from your head. People were happily popping pills. The medical establishment was basking in its own glory. We were mapping the entire human genome, which promised solutions for all kinds of health problems. Who needed Wellness when *Medicine* was responsible for our health?

*Paul Zane Pilzer, *The Wellness Revolution*, John Wiley & Sons, Inc., ©2002.

A decade later, the term *Wellness* is found in books, the mass media, and even in scientific journals. The popular press is finally reporting the astronomical numbers of deaths due to medications and other medical mishaps. The Human Genome Project was completed, with damning results. Rather than the roughly 140,000 genes required to explain human life, only about 30,000 were found. We have barely more genes than a fruit fly. So much for genetic determinism! People are beginning to realize that pills and potions are not the answer for a healthy, fulfilling life. In fact, we now know that pharmaceuticals are a leading *cause* of death and health problems. And many medical principles that were gospel just 10 years ago have now been debunked.

Prior to the Baby Boomer generation, people were happy to simply survive. Health was measured in terms of *lifespan.* Due to poor sanitation, a lack of personal and community hygiene, malnutrition, and difficult living conditions, people died from diseases that spread like wildfire through community after community. Surviving to 60 was considered a victory.

Due to improvements in hygiene and standard-of-living, along with medical advancements such as antibiotics, we largely ended the scourge of early deaths due to infectious diseases. During the 20th Century, life expectancy skyrocketed. People now commonly live into their 70's, 80's, and 90's.

But this did not come without a price. Chronic conditions such as cancer, heart disease, and diabetes also skyrocketed, as did arthritic conditions. In addition, medications became popular for *all* health conditions, not just the life-threatening ones. Overuse of these medications has led to an epidemic of iatrogenic (caused by medicine) illness and deaths. According to some sources, Medicine has overtaken heart disease as the leading cause of death in America!

There was a second tragic consequence. Since certain medicines significantly reduced death rates due to infectious diseases, the Medical Establishment became idolized. People looked to Medicine for answers to all sorts of health conditions. Medicine was happy to oblige. And happy to create a multi-trillion dollar industry. Because of this false sense of security, our culture became extremely irresponsible with our lifestyle choices. And today, a frightening number of Americans turn to psychotropic prescription drugs to numb their minds, rather than face the challenges of their lives.

Medicine has proven to be a very poor solution for the illnesses and conditions we now face. Despite their best efforts and trillions of research dollars, Medicine has failed to produce answers to heart disease, cancer, diabetes, arthritis, and other common conditions. More people die from heart attacks than ever before. While the survival rates for certain cancers have somewhat improved, we still use the same basic treatments as we did 40 years ago—chemotherapy and radiation. It is estimated that more than one-third of all children born today will become diabetic. Arthritis and pain drugs have been recently linked to tens of thousands of deaths. Over half of all deaths over the age of 70 are linked to *medications*, not natural causes.

What's even more troubling is the significant decline in our quality of life. In other words, we now have more years in our life, but less life in our years. As a culture we are obese, exhausted, depressed and drugged out. While the medical establishment deserves their share of credit for our increased lifespan, it also deserves much of the blame for our pathetic state of health.

Today, people are looking for something different, something better. Baby Boomers have seen their parents wither away in nursing homes, or struggle with the adverse physical and mental effects of the many medications they have been prescribed. They don't want to end up in this situation themselves. So they are looking outside Medicine for answers. They dance to the oldies, buy retro cars, join health clubs, and get face-lifts—all with the desired result of youth and vitality.

But where do you find the "Fountain of Youth"? Where can you get a "prescription" for this thing called Wellness? For more than 100 years, chiropractors and their patients have shared an idea called the "Chiropractic Lifestyle" with family, friends, and others. By maintaining a healthy spine and a properly functioning nervous system, by making healthy lifestyle choices, and by avoiding drugs and surgeries except as a last resort, this subculture has experienced a youthful vigor and quality of life that others can only dream of.

But a culture dominated by the promise of quick fixes and miracle cures was not ready to hear this message. Chiropractors and their healthy clients were relegated to the fringe of our massive healthcare system. That is, until NOW.

What is Wellness?

Wellness can be defined as a high level of life experience. Chiropractors speak of life expression and human potential. Wellness is a state where humans express their full life potential. Wellness is a state of balance, bliss, and satisfaction achieved through an outstanding quality of life. When you see someone who has it all together—physically, mentally, emotionally, socially, spiritually, and financially—you are viewing a snapshot of Wellness.

Sickness is the opposite of Wellness. The 20th century was dominated by an obsessive focus on sickness. Germs were the enemy. Drugs were king. Our body was something to fear. We were told that our health was determined by our genes—a lie that created a perfect excuse to be irresponsible. The 21st century will be dominated by a focus on Wellness. A time to restore a healthy respect for our body's ability to heal and self-regulate—with a limited need for dangerous drugs. This marks a new era of **personal responsibility**, a realization that only we can heal ourselves.

Wellness is *not* the same as what Medicine has termed "prevention". Preventive Medicine is an oxymoron. The idea of taking enough tests until we find something "wrong", or using drugs to replace healthy habits and the body's innate ability to heal is ridiculous. It's like slashing your tires to reduce fuel consumption. It may work as advertised, but it creates a bigger mess than it solves.

4 Steps To Wellness

There are many components of Wellness which will be discussed throughout this book. Physical Fitness, Emotional Wellness, Physical Health, Proper Nervous System Function, Financial Wellness, Spiritual Wellness, Quality Sleep, Nutrition, and Social Wellness are all part of our life and being. In each area, there are 4 steps required to improve your quality of life.

Step 1. Make A Decision

Nothing ever changes unless you first make a decision. The reason most people fail is that they never really decide in the first place.

Once you decide that something absolutely, positively must change, you have navigated the largest single obstacle to change.

Step 2. Get Informed

Once you have decided to make a change, learn how. This book is a how-to guide for lifelong Wellness. There are thousands of other resources and references available, including the chiropractor who provided this book.

Step 3. Take Action

It makes no difference what you decide or what you know until you take action. In fact, many experts claim that someone hasn't really decided until they act on that decision.

Step 4. Stay The Course

The secret to improvement in any area of life is consistent action. Many of your choices will meet with resistance from others. These people may include your family, friends, or even your medical doctor. It is up to you to stand behind your decisions, no matter what others may say or how difficult the road may be.

That's it! There is no magic formula, just consistent work on the multiple areas of your Wellness. If you are wise, you are ready for this new paradigm. A way of life that promotes healing from within, healthy lifestyle choices, and limiting the use of harmful medications. If you have been searching for a better way to live, this book is for you. By using the ideas and tools in this book, you will have the opportunity to expand your life in many dimensions. By utilizing Chiropractic to maintain a healthy spine and nervous system, and utilizing this book to create a healthier lifestyle, you can achieve the life of your dreams.

Exercise

Make a list of *Wellness Opportunities*. These are things that you now do (or know you *could* do) to improve your health and Wellness.

Chapter 2

Are We More Than A Machine?

mechanism—1. a machine or machine-like structure. 3. the theory that the phenomena of life are based on the same physical and chemical laws which operate in the inorganic [non-living] world; opposed to *vitalism.*

Vitalism—the theory, opposed to *mechanism*, that biological activities are due to a vital force or principle distinct from physical and chemical forces.

***Dorland's Medical Dictionary*, 28th Edition**

This chapter begins with two definitions taken directly from *Dorland's Medical Dictionary*. Read them again. The theory of *Mechanism* clearly states that living things are no different than non-living things. That at our essence, human beings are no different than rocks. The human *being* is regarded as a mere *machine*. **By its very definition, *Mechanism* denies the existence of God or any intelligent, creative force in the process of life!**

This explanation of life falls somewhere between extremely limited and downright outrageous. After all, we don't see water grow arms or rocks suddenly jump in the air. It is plain old common sense that there is some force, some intelligence, that separates the living from the non-living. But did you know that *Mechanism* is the foundational theory for the entire field of Medicine?

Virtually every field of science has replaced Newtonian (mechanistic) physics with the new and significantly improved Quantum Physics. That is, except Medicine. While *Mechanism* can accurately describe the orbit of the earth around the sun and what happens when you mix an acid with a base, it is woefully unable to explain the miracle of *life*.

Why has Medicine stubbornly refused to update its basic theory of life? One reason is that every medical theory, teaching, and treatment is based upon *Mechanism*! To admit this error would mean rethinking and rewriting *all* medical theories. Yes, there are times when the mechanisms of the body need assistance beyond what nature can provide. However, admitting that the fundamental medical principle was *wrong* would expose the failed attempts of Medicine to create the health and Wellness they have promised for decades.

The second reason is this. Medicine would have to admit that holistic healing arts such as Chiropractic and naturopathy (professions that Medicine has forever condemned as "unscientific") were actually right all along! Up until this point in history, it has been professional suicide for anyone within the medical establishment to give credit to any person or concept contrary to medical doctrine. But as a stunning amount of research accumulates, more and more medical professionals are opening their eyes to the truth.

Unlike *Mechanism*, which denies the existence of a vital force or intelligence, *Vitalism* accepts the existence of chemistry and physics. However, *Vitalism* states that these mechanisms are controlled by a vital force or intelligence.

This theory is not only sensible, but it has been proven true by a large body of scientific research. As one example, there have been numerous scientific studies on distant prayer. These studies have demonstrated that people who are prayed for have significantly higher survival rates and shorter healing time. Without *Vitalism*, these findings would be impossible.

Chiropractic and other holistic healing arts are based on *Vitalism*. It is for this reason alone that these non-medical approaches to health have been at various times labeled as "unscientific", "religions", "charlatans", and worse by members of the medical profession. How ironic!

Chiropractic principles were true all along. It simply took decades for *science* to catch up with *philosophy*. There are many other differences between Medicine and Chiropractic. To know the difference between a life powered by nature and a life dictated by chemistry, you must understand these differences.

Chiropractic	**Medicine**
Natural	Artificial
Holistic	Reductionistic
Humanistic	Authoritarian
Cause-Oriented	Symptom-Based

Medicine is **Artificial**. Medicine distrusts nature. In fact, Medicine's primary objective is to *fool* nature by altering natural processes. One of the major mistakes the medical profession has made is their false (and arrogant) belief that doctors and scientists are smarter than Mother Nature.

Chiropractic is **Natural.** It relies on natural and universal laws and principles. A Wellness lifestyle trusts in nature's wisdom.

Medicine is **Reductionistic**. This is the belief that the human body is simply the sum of a number of independent parts. Medicine adds chemicals or subtracts parts, ignoring the fact that every part of the body works together as an entire system.

Chiropractic is **Holistic.** In other words, *the whole is far greater than the parts.* Chiropractors care for the whole person, not a single part, condition, or symptom.

Medicine is **Authoritarian**. This is defined as favoring blind submission to authority and favoring concentration of power in a leader or an elite not constitutionally responsible to the people. Could anything be more true? Medicine despises anyone (patient, family member, scientist, or medical professional) that dares question their absolute power. This occurs on an individual level, as patients are threatened, chastised, or ridiculed for asking questions. It occurs on a professional level, as the medical profession attacks other healing arts and even medical doctors who have differing views. It happens on a cultural level, as the media is filled with propaganda designed to create fear and provide grandiose promises of miracle cures. The medical profession has used its authoritarian power for political gain by manipulating laws and using government agencies to destroy individual freedoms.

Chiropractic is **Humanistic**. In this sense, Wellness professionals stress *the individual's dignity, worth, and capacity for self-realization*. Chiropractors believe in the importance of education, and cherish opportunities to help clients realize their own tremendous gifts and abilities. Chiropractors believe that people should make their own decisions, based on what is right for *them*.

Medicine is **Symptom-Based**. In other words, medicine views the symptom *as* the disease. There are many medical treatments that offer effective *short-term* relief from symptoms. The problem with this approach is that it solves nothing, and often creates bigger long-term problems. When you have a stomach ache, you get a pill for your stomach. When your gall bladder creates discomfort, it gets taken out. If you have allergies, you get an allergy pill. If you have hypertension, you get a high blood pressure pill. If you are depressed, you get a depression pill. If you have anxiety, you get an anxiety pill (basically the opposite of a depression pill). If your child is bored or overly creative, you give them a sit still and be quiet pill. If the sit still and be quiet pill keeps them from sleeping, they get a sleeping pill. If you have headaches, you take a headache pill. Never once does the doctor ask "Why?"

Chiropractic is **Cause-Oriented**. Chiropractors always ask "Why?" The only way to restore health in any meaningful way is to find the true cause of a condition or interference to health. Rather than simply treating a headache with a drug, chiropractors want to discover why that particular client is having the symptom of headaches. Rather than vainly attempting to "cure" a digestive problem, a chiropractor looks for the cause. Is it nerve interference? Is something in the diet contributing to the problem? Is it a medication? Is there something stressful in the client's life that is manifesting in this condition? Is it a lack of exercise and activity? *Chiropractors see symptoms as the solution to health problems.*

Is a headache caused by a lack of aspirin? Is high blood pressure caused by a lack of a diuretic? Is constipation caused by a lack of Ex-Lax? Is depression caused by a lack of Prozac? Is a child's high level of activity, creativity, and curiosity caused by a lack of Ritalin? Is the flu caused by a lack of a cocktail of mercury, aluminum and viruses? Of course not! But the pharmaceutical industry spends billions of dollars trying to convince you that they are. And these are all standard medical protocols!

Exercise

Which of the following best fits your personal beliefs regarding life and health?

A. Living things posses a vital intelligence which makes them different from non-living things. *Or*

B. Life can be fully explained and controlled through chemistry and physics.

A. We may not fully understand how it works, but Mother Nature usually knows best. *Or*

B. Nature is something to fear. The body is broken, something we need to "fix".

A. The human body, as a whole system, is greater than the sum of its parts. *Or*

B. We can explain everything that happens in the body simply by looking at each individual part.

A. Health relates to the person. Everyone should make the choices and decisions which are right for them. *Or*

B. We should always do what the doctor says. We should never question the need for or adverse effects of treatments. Doctors and government should dictate our health care.

A. We should always look to correct the *underlying cause* of symptoms or conditions, not just the symptoms or conditions themselves. It is important to promote health within the body in order to prevent future symptoms or conditions. *Or*

B. The primary purpose of health care is to minimize or eliminate symptoms.

Total number of A's __________ B's __________

How many A's did you circle? How many B's? If you have mostly A's, your philosophy and beliefs are closely aligned with Chiropractic and the Wellness paradigm. If most of your answers were B, your beliefs and philosophy are closely aligned with Medicine. If you have an even mix of A's and B's, your beliefs and philosophy fall somewhere between Wellness and allopathic medicine.

So, if you believe that your body is no more intelligent than a rock, that your genes hold your fate, that the best way to be healthy is to artificially alter your body function, and that you should take what your doctor says as gospel, then your beliefs closely match those held by medicine. It will be a challenge for you to adopt a Wellness lifestyle, unless you create a shift in your belief systems.

But if you believe that life is a gift from God, that you are fully equipped to adapt to most stresses in your life, that you should handle health naturally whenever possible, that you should always ask questions about all recommendations from any health professional, and that ultimately you are in control of and responsible for your health and vitality, then your beliefs align perfectly with the Chiropractic Wellness paradigm. The more you learn about the tremendous potential inside of you, the more motivated you will become to live the life of your dreams.

Chapter 3

Chiropractic—The Foundation Of Wellness

A Tale Of Two Sons

This is a story of my two sons, born nine years apart, and born into two completely different philosophies of health. It is also the story of two very different forms of health care.

The first is a politically, economically, and socially powerful approach that few have questioned, even though its shortcomings and dangers have become increasingly obvious.

The second is an approach that has survived and is beginning to thrive not because of political power or social pressures, but for one reason only—the tremendous results it has produced in the lives of people willing to live life at a higher level.

Bryan was born on January 19, 1996 in the midst of a Wisconsin snowstorm. Perhaps this was foreshadowing, because nothing in his early life went well. While his mother and I were extremely joyful about the pregnancy and the anticipation of our first child, Valerie had a miserable pregnancy.

The truth is, she was actually sick *before* the pregnancy, even though we thought that asthma, allergies, a weak immune system, and a constant lack of energy were pretty much *normal.* We had been told that it was. Our friends, families, and co-workers had many similar health problems. The stories we saw over and over again in the media explained that most people were doomed to be sick because of their genetics and other uncontrollable factors.

We heard again and again that our only hope to save the human race was the amazing and magical field of Medicine, which bragged endlessly about all of their cures and other accomplishments, and promised even more cures—for AIDS, cancer, heart disease, and diabetes—even for that nasty fungus that people get under their toenails. Scientists were coming close to mapping the entire human genome. Once they did, we could find a genetic cure for practically everything. If only given enough time and money, our doctors and researchers would find an answer for all that ails us!

Almost immediately after becoming pregnant, Valerie had severe morning sickness. The medicines she was taking for her other symptoms began making her feel miserable. She began having premature labor at five months and was placed on bed rest by her sixth month. She later confided in me that, as much as she wanted to have a child, she really hated being pregnant.

Valerie went into full labor three weeks before her due date. Since Bryan was in a breech position, a C-section was performed. Although somewhat small (5 1/2 lbs.) and 3 weeks early, Bryan appeared perfectly normal to all of the doctors, and his initial APGAR tests were relatively normal. After the delivery, Valerie was immediately put on high doses of pain medications, which made her extremely groggy. This was kept up for **three days.** To this day, she hardly remembers anything about her hospital stay.

We returned home after three miserable days in the hospital. I still remember the big bunch of blue balloons sitting on the dining room table and how proud and excited we were as new parents. But challenges arose immediately. Bryan had difficulty nursing, and would only feed on one side. The nurse blamed this on Valerie, chastising her mothering ability, and told us to put the baby on formula immediately. This furthered the nursing problems, to the point that Bryan was on full formula within 5 weeks.

After Bryan returned from his first "Well-baby" visit, Valerie was visibly upset. Even though Bryan was low birth weight and premature (two significant contraindications for vaccination), the doctors gave him all of his "Well-Baby shots". Then, they proceeded to add hepatitis B vaccine (even though we had **no** risk for hepatitis B in our family) and chicken pox (a "voluntary" vaccine) without ever asking for consent. Bryan screamed all day and all night, broke out in a pox-like rash, and ran a 105° fever for five days. When we called the pediatrician, we were told this was a "normal reaction", that there was no need to worry, and that we should give Bryan acetaminophen for the fever.

By the time Bryan was a month old, he had never slept longer than two hours at a time. He spit up and threw up constantly. He was fussy and cried pretty much all the time. We thought this was just the way babies were—after all, the doctors didn't seem too concerned. We were given medicines for the colic and told to try different formulas to find one that he didn't throw up.

When Bryan received his second set of "Well-Baby" shots, he became extremely irritable (even more than usual) and ran a 105° fever for several days. We were concerned about the post-vaccination pattern showing up, but were again reassured by the pediatricians that this was a normal reaction to the vaccinations and we were just "over-concerned parents".

When Bryan was six months old, he had still never slept more than two hours at a time—ever. He was still having trouble keeping formula down. He was not growing as quickly as he should. His motor skills and development were lagging way behind. Something wasn't right. We just didn't know what it was.

Apparently, neither did the doctors. We were given more medications for the colic, which hadn't improved from the first drugs. We were also told by leading pediatricians that Bryan would never be normal, that the C-section was somehow affecting his brain, and he needed to get a full set of skull x-rays, MRIs, and a visit to a neurologist for a surgical consult. When we refused this invasive, ridiculous "let's hope we get lucky and find something" approach, we were promptly visited at our home by Child Protective Services since we had refused "necessary" medical attention.

At his third "Well-Baby" visit, we expressed concerns over his previous reactions to the vaccines. We were told not to worry, these were *normal reactions that the doctors saw very frequently*. And then we were told we didn't have a choice because Bryan "won't be allowed in school without all of his shots."

Bryan had a nearly constant high-pitched squeal the first night after his third "Well-Baby" visit. Then, he basically laid in his crib, hardly fed, and ran a fever for the next week. On the sixth day, Valerie became frightened when Bryan's blue eyes began to roll back into his head. When she called the clinic to report this, she was abruptly told that there was "absolutely, positively no chance that this had anything to do with the vaccines." It was at this point that we, as parents, decided that we would no longer rely on the judgment of the medical profession. We were being lied to. We needed a different approach.

As is the way with the universe, not two weeks later we "bumped into" a chiropractor at a local health fair. Without our even saying a word, she asked about Bryan's health. She said that she noticed a problem in the way he carried his head and neck, which could affect the normal flow of nerve signals. I had utilized Chiropractic since the age of 12, but always for a specific pain or symptom. It had never dawned on me that a chiropractor could help someone so young. After a visit to her office for a thorough history and exam, she recommended a series of Chiropractic adjustments to correct the problem in Bryan's upper neck and some gentle techniques to help the cranial plates move to a more normal position.

Within one month of care, Bryan was sleeping through the night, his colic permanently resolved, and his development began to catch up. He began smiling. By the time Bryan was 12 months old, he was perfectly normal and perfectly healthy.*

In the eight years since, Bryan has taken **no** medications. No foreign substances have been injected into his precious body. Other than a couple of very mild colds, he has not shown a single sign of ill health since. He doesn't have allergies. He doesn't have asthma. He hasn't even had more than a terribly minor cold or sniffles. He asks us to tuck him in between 8:00 and 8:30 every night, falls asleep immediately, sleeps all night, wakes up at 6:30, and is non-stop action from 6:30 in the morning to 8:00 at night. Every day! He is extremely athletic, smart and sociable. A far cry from the sick child the medics promised us!

Here's the kicker. When we recently reviewed copies of Bryan's medical records, there was **no mention whatsoever** of his multiple adverse reactions to vaccinations! But there **is** a record of our "irresponsible" parenting

*I am eternally grateful to Dr. Lisa Turek-Shay, D.C., Amery, Wisconsin for changing the course of Bryan's life forever and for opening my eyes to the incredible healing power of the chiropractic adjustment.

because we refused "important medical intervention". Many parents make the mistake of asking their pediatrician about Chiropractic for their child. Without any scientific basis to back it up, many pediatricians simply read off a whole list of baloney and tell the parent why a child should never ever see a chiropractor! This is like asking a urologist if you should see a dentist.

Bryan was our first child. His life began in the world of Medicine. His life was transformed by the world of Chiropractic. The incredible changes we saw in Bryan's life convinced me to dedicate my life to helping others. I returned to college to become a chiropractor myself. Now I get to see miracles like Bryan's every day.

Our second son, Brendan, was born nine years and 12 days after Bryan. Our life is quite different now. Through the power of Chiropractic and the Chiropractic lifestyle, Valerie has gone from severely ill to totally 100% healthy. Our philosophy of health and our lifestyle choices have also changed dramatically.

Valerie went through nine months of pregnancy without a single health problem. No morning sickness. No nausea. No premature labor. No depression. No need to change her regular activities. Perhaps this was because *she* was now healthy.

Brendan was born at 9:12 pm on February 1, 2005. He received his first Chiropractic adjustment one hour later. All of his vitals remained perfect every time he was checked. Brendan began nursing almost immediately. When we returned home, he was already sleeping 3–4 hours at a time.

Brendan received no vaccines or medications. The only foreign substance he received was a preservative-free vitamin K shot. He is checked for subluxation frequently, and gets adjusted about three times per week.

From the time of his birth to the time of this writing, Brendan has *never* spit up or thrown up. He sleeps from about 7:00 pm to 2:00 am, nurses and falls back asleep from about 3:00 to 7:00. He has never had a sniffle or anything resembling illness. He loves the fine art on our walls and his favorite TV show is American Idol—he laughs and smiles when the contestants sing, then gets angry and fussy when they stop! He loves watching sports, except he gets a little frustrated because he can't run.

Brendan can reach for and grab his toys, and clearly forms and says the words "Hello" and "OK" to everyone. **One day** after his mom started playing peek-a-boo with him, he began pulling the blanket over his face and now plays peek-a-boo by himself! He is extremely aware with big, bright eyes that constantly dart back and forth across the room observing everything. He has learned to walk with minimal assistance. None of this would be remarkable, except Brendan is three months old!

These two very different stories have nothing to do with luck, or genetics, or any of the other excuses the medical profession has blamed for our declining health. This is a true story about two distinctly different philosophies and approaches to health.

The first has used its political, economic, and social power to overreach its own abilities. The second has relied only on its tremendous results and outcomes to create a small but growing subculture of truly healthy people. This is a story about a failing *medical* system and a growing *Wellness* system, with Chiropractic in the leading role.

Our children desperately need our help. Their lives hang in the balance. We all share responsibility in ending the current insanity in order to give our kids the opportunity to live healthy and fulfilling lives.

Chiropractic 101

Chiropractic is the largest natural primary health care profession in the world. Although largely misunderstood, it has produced the most remarkable results of any health care discipline—both in terms of personal experiences and in the scientific literature. Doctors of Chiropractic and their patients have long known the far-reaching benefits of Chiropractic care, and recent advances in research are beginning to show more and more scientific evidence of these benefits.

To understand Chiropractic, you must have a basic understanding of how your body functions. At the time of your conception, your Inner Wisdom knew exactly how to take two cells and create a fully functioning human being. From the time you were born, this same intelligence has known exactly how to keep you alive and healthy. Chiropractors call this inborn wisdom *Innate Intelligence.* Your Innate Intelligence is what makes your heart beat about 70 times a minute, *every minute of your life.* It also tells your heart to beat faster if you are exercising or preparing for a physical challenge. Innate controls your breathing, your digestion, your immune system, your hormones and blood chemistry, your body temperature, and your blood pressure. In fact, there are millions of details every second of your life that require the careful guidance of Innate Intelligence. This is the same higher intelligence that medical treatments ignore.

Your Innate Intelligence is distributed throughout your body by a complex Information Superhighway called the Nervous System. According to *Gray's Anatomy,* your Nervous System is responsible for **all other body functions.** Every second of every day. Just as your skull protects your brain, your spine protects your spinal cord and other vital parts of your nervous system. Your spine also sends millions of nerve signals per second to the brain. When your spine loses its proper alignment or motion, the normal pattern of nerve signals flowing throughout your body is disturbed. This prevents your Innate Intelligence from guiding and regulating body processes. This disturbance is called a *Subluxation.*

Chemical and emotional stresses can also lead to subluxation. These include things such as diet, chemical additives, environmental toxins and pollutants, medications, other drugs, and life issues.

Subluxations need not be painful to be devastating. Even small disturbances, over time, can significantly alter body processes, leading to a significant threat to your health. Studies have demonstrated that even a minimal amount of pressure placed on nerves where they exit the spine is enough to reduce their function by 40–60%.

The primary role your chiropractor serves is to remove nerve interference and restore the normal flow of Innate Intelligence. This allows your body to return to its natural state of health and healing. This type of healing is not completed in a single visit, which is why your chiropractor will typically recommend a series of visits—to give ample time for your body to support the changes made. Once your health is restored, you would be wise to join a rapidly growing number of Chiropractic clients who opt for Wellness care—to continue to improve your health and quality of life. In fact, if your health and well-being are so dependant on the function of your spine and nervous system, why would you *ever* want to stop receiving the many benefits of Chiropractic care?

Subluxations, or nerve interference, are corrected primarily through *Chiropractic adjustments.* An adjustment is **not** the same as making your neck pop or an M.D. giving a "manipulation". An adjustment is a carefully applied, specific input of energy into the spine and nervous system intended to improve function within your nervous system, brain, and body. Chiropractors spend years mastering the art of adjusting.

M.D.'s and physical therapists typically take weekend courses in "manipulation" and simply twist or push on the spine to get some sort of audible movement. They falsely assume that this is the same as an adjustment. Some osteopaths are sufficiently qualified in "osteopathic manipulation". But again, this is *not* the same as a chiropractic adjustment. Just as only cardiologists are qualified to do heart surgery, only chiropractors are qualified to remove nerve interference through spinal adjustments.

Chiropractors use a number of different techniques to restore normal nerve function. Some use their hands to physically move a vertebra, often resulting in an audible release of pressure and tension from the joints. Others use tools specifically designed for spinal adjustments. Still others use non-force techniques. All accepted Chiropractic techniques are very safe and effective.

Exercise

Think about the following questions:

How does your blood know when to clot? When *not* to clot?

How does your body know how and when to mend a broken bone?

How does your heart know to beat faster when you are running? Or when you see a vicious dog running toward you?

Why do you begin to salivate—when you've only *smelled* the food?

How does your body maintain the appropriate levels of blood sugar, hormones and digestive enzymes?

How does your immune system know to attack foreign invaders (even those it's never "seen" before)? How does it know to attack cancer cells but not healthy cells?

How does your body know that harmful pathogens die at temps above 100°F and have the intelligence to create a fever?

What Chiropractic *Is* and What Chiropractic *Is Not*

A major reason for the misunderstandings and misrepresentations of Chiropractic is the attempt to define *Chiropractic* in *medical* terms. Medicine focuses on the idea of *cure*, which means something outside the body eliminating a disease or symptom. However, Chiropractic does not work in terms of cure. It works in terms of *healing*.

Chiropractic is NOT a cure for ANY medical disease, symptom, or diagnosis. The sole intention of Chiropractic is to remove interference to the nervous system, thus restoring the Innate ability to heal and self regulate. The ultimate goal of Chiropractic care is to return the WHOLE PERSON to their NATURAL STATE OF HEALTH.

Doctors of Chiropractic are stuck between a rock and a hard place in attempting to explain or justify what they do. People *do* seek the services of a chiropractor for *a wide variety* of health conditions. Then, when the condition improves or goes away, the patient tells their family, friends, everyone they know (often including their medical doctor) that their chiropractor *cured* them of their particular condition. **It is vital to understand that when conditions or symptoms improve or resolve as a result of Chiropractic care, it is your own body that has done the *healing*. The chiropractor simply removed the interference that had been preventing you from healing all along.**

To bring this point home, let me share a case that occurred recently in my practice. On March 30, 2005, L. E. came to my office complaining of lower back and neck pain. We did the normal nerve testing, examination and took full spine Chiropractic x-rays. The computerized nerve testing, the exam, and the x-rays all pointed to two subluxations—one in her neck and one in her sacrum (tailbone). I adjusted both places, and she returned home. Due to financial issues, she was unable to return for follow-up care until 1 month later. She was experiencing mild discomfort in the same two areas.

When she walked into the adjusting room, she practically beamed as she shared with me her experience. "When I came in last month, I was having another problem that I didn't even mention, because I didn't see how you could help it. Since the birth of my child two years ago, I have suffered from severe constipation and hemorrhoids. I have seen five medical doctors, all of whom gave me medications that didn't do anything. But within one day after my adjustment, the constipation went away and *I haven't had any problem with either my bowels or my hemorrhoids since!*"

While I was obviously pleased, I was careful to make two things clear to L.E. First, while we see miracles every day, her immediate and total improvement was unusual. Typically it takes more time for the body to produce that kind of a change. Second, *it was her own inner healing capacity that produced the change.* I simply removed interference to her body's controlling mechanism, which allowed her body to function exactly the way it was supposed to.

Chiropractic patients have experienced remarkable results for a number of different health conditions. This is not because Chiropractic "cured" their symptoms or condition. Rather, it's because Chiropractic returned them to a place where their body could heal—the way nature intended.

Over time, Chiropractic care commonly produces the following and other results: Reduced pain, Reduced symptoms, Improved organ functions, Fewer chronic conditions, Slowing of the aging and degenerative processes, Less reliance on drugs and surgeries, Increased energy levels, Improved sleep, Increased flexibility, Improved ability to perform activities, Improved mental clarity, Improved emotional health, Stronger immune system, Greater resistance to disease, Improved coordination and athletic performance, Improved sense of well-being.

Recent chiropractic research has focused more on chiropractic's effects on internal and cellular function. Research demonstrates that Chiropractic may have a profound effect on such things as DNA damage and repair (actually slows the aging process of genes), HIV/AIDS, the immune system, and the inflammatory process (a well-known factor in chronic diseases and conditions).*

Chiropractic Is NOT "Alternative Medicine"

As is typically the case, Medicine has proclaimed *itself* the "real" health care system. Therefore, they proclaim any health care profession *not* Medicine to be "alternative". Again, we have a situation where the arrogant medical establishment defines Chiropractic in medical terms!

* References can be found at the end of this chapter.

Chiropractic is a separate and distinct art, science and philosophy of health. It has nothing whatsoever to do with Medicine. In fact, the powerful medical industry has made every conceivable attempt to eliminate the Chiropractic profession over the past 100 years. Why? Because Chiropractic offers a completely different model of health that threatens the medical establishment's total authority!

Chiropractic is an alternative *to* Medicine. This doesn't mean that people can't utilize both Chiropractic and allopathic medicine. In a perfect world, everyone would utilize both systems at the appropriate times. The Wellness Paradigm does not suggest or recommend that we altogether avoid or eliminate allopathic medicine. It simply means that we only utilize medical approaches in crises or emergencies, or when safer natural approaches are unable to solve a problem. Wellness-based disciplines and sickness-based (allopathic) disciplines would *share* responsibility. Perhaps this is what the medical establishment is afraid of.

In a perfect world, Medicine would focus on its *strengths*—trauma, emergencies, fractures, immediate life-threatening illnesses, life-threatening infectious diseases, genetic disorders, *complicated* pregnancy/ delivery, and conditions which are unresponsive to safer approaches.

All other health and Wellness needs **would *first* be addressed by more conservative, natural approaches and through lifestyle management.**

This world may be a long way off. The medical establishment simply has too much power to give up their stranglehold over our nation's healthcare delivery system. However you, your family, and your friends *can* make this change immediately! The choice is yours. Look around you. Are you comfortable with the status of our current symptom-based system? Are you willing to just sit around and wait for something bad to happen? If not, the first decision you can make is to join the millions of Americans living the Wellness Lifestyle. There *are* safe, effective, and *scientifically valid* alternatives to drugs and surgeries for you and your family.

How Does Chiropractic Work?

When M.D.'s and others look at Chiropractic through their Mechanistic lens, it is often difficult for them to understand how a spinal adjustment can impact the entire body, mind, and overall health and function. This doesn't make Chiropractic any less scientific- it simply points out how difficult it is to learn a "foreign language."

There has never before been such astonishing scientific research which proves the validity of Chiropractic. At the same time that research has called into question the most closely held medical beliefs, studies are demonstrating Chiropractic benefits on a cellular and even DNA level! A significant amount of research now demonstrates the intimate relationship between the nervous system and cellular function. There is no question that the nervous system is closely intertwined with both the immune system and endocrine (hormone) system. In fact, we now know that these three systems, previously thought to be separate, talk to each other on a moment-by-moment basis. *There is no doubt that the most important protector and predictor of health is the nervous system.*

While we may never know the full impact that the chiropractic adjustment has on the nervous system, there are several effects that we do know of. Here are just a few of many:

- Nerve Compression. In the state of subluxation, nerve tissues (notably the *nerve root*) can be stretched, chaffed, compressed, or otherwise irritated by bone, disc, muscles, ligaments, or other soft tissues. In this case, adjustments help reduce the direct compression or irritation to nerve tissue.
- Spinal Cord Distortion. In the state of subluxation, offending vertebrae can alter the spinal cord, either directly or through ligaments that line the spinal canal. Again in this case, adjustments reduce direct interference to the normal flow of nerve signals.
- Altered Nerve Reflexes. We are talking about the millions of internal reflexes contained in our nervous system, not just the muscular ones. In the state of subluxation, these reflexes, which control and maintain vital life functions, are disturbed. Adjustments serve to break faulty reflex patterns, allowing them to return to a more normal state.
- Local Inflammatory Response. In subluxation, mechanical breakdown of spinal joint and muscle function can

create acute or chronic inflammation. Nerves are extremely sensitive to inflammatory chemicals. In this case, adjustments correct the underlying mechanical disturbance, reducing the amount of local inflammation.

- Disturbed Cerebrospinal Fluid Flow. Subluxation can disturb the normal flow of cerebrospinal fluid up and down the spinal cord and through the brain. This "stasis" causes a lack of nutrients and a buildup of toxins, affecting the entire nervous system. In this case, adjustments help restore normal cerebrospinal respiration.
- Altered Circulation. In subluxation, circulation to the spinal cord and nerve roots can be compromised, leading to a loss of nerve function. In this case, adjustments help restore normal blood supply to nerve tissue.

But perhaps the major effect of adjustments on the nervous system (and therefore all parts of the body and all aspects of health) is through *afferent input*. This area of neurology is just beginning to be fully researched, with remarkable recent discoveries.

- Altered Afferent Input. Afferent input is nerve signals traveling *from* the body *to* the spinal cord and brain. Every second, millions of nerve signals travel from the spine and body, up the spinal cord, and to the appropriate regions of the brain. This information is vital, as it give the brain input regarding the health status of the entire body. In the state of subluxation, faulty spinal alignment and movements send faulty input to the brain, creating a false perception of the body. This causes the *brain itself* to adopt an unhealthy pattern of activity, sending unhealthy instructions back to the body. This also affects our ability to think and our emotional health. By restoring normal spinal alignment and motion patterns (and direct input into the nervous system), adjustments improve the quality and pattern of nerve signals traveling to the brain.

It is a scientific fact that the nervous system controls every aspect of our thoughts, senses, and body function. It is also a fact that Chiropractic adjustments improve and maintain the quality of information traveling through the brain, spinal cord, and nerves. While it is impossible to predict the exact benefits that an individual will receive through Chiropractic, it is an indisputable fact that Chiropractic adjustments help to restore function, assist the healing process, and promote Wellness.

References:

Campbell CJ, Kent C, Banne A, Amiri A, Pero RW: Surrogate Indication of DNA Repair in Serum After Long Term Chiropractic Intervention – A Retrospective Study. *Journal of Vertebral Subluxation Research* February 18, 2005, pp 1-5.

Owen DE, Rix GDW: The effect of chiropractic manipulation on serum levels of immunoglobulin M. *European Journal of Chiropractic* 2002;48:55.

Davison, S, Parkin-Smith GF: The possible effect of upper cervical chiropractic manipulation on short-term lymphocytic response: a pilot study. *European Journal of Chiropractic* 2003;51:19.

Kaminski TM: Female infertility and chiropractic wellness care: a case study on the autonomic nervous system response while under subluxation based chiropractic care and subsequent fertility. *Journal of Vertebral Subluxation Research* 2003.

Behrendt M, Olsen N: The impact of subluxation correction on mental health: reduction of anxiety in a female patient under chiropractic care. *Journal of Vertebral Subluxation Research* 2003.

Takeda Y, Arai S, Touichi H: Long Term remission and alleviation of Crohn' Disease in patients following spinal adjustments for reduction of vertebral subluxations. *Journal of Vertebral Subluxation Research* 2002;4(4);129.

Yun AJ, Lee PY, Bazar KA: Autonomic dysregulation as a basis of cardiovascular, endocrine, and inflammatory disturbances associated with sleep apnea and other conditions of chronic hypoxia, hypercapnia, and acidosis. *Medical Hypotheses* 2004;62(6):852.

Elster EL: Eighty-one patients with multiple sclerosis and Parkinson's disease undergoing upper cervical chiropractic care to correct vertebral subluxation: a retrospective analysis. *Journal of Vertebral Subluxation Research* 2003.

Winsor H: Sympathetic segmental disturbances—II. The evidences of the association, in dissected cadavers, of visceral disease with vertebral deformities of the same sympathetic segments. *The Medical Times* November 1921, pp. 267-271.

Author's note: These are but a small few of the many studies demonstrating the effects of chiropractic care on visceral and cellular health and function.

Chiropractic Principles

The Power That Made The Body Heals The Body.

All Living Things Possess An Inborn Wisdom Called Innate Intelligence.

Innate Intelligence Is That Creative Energy Which Allows Us To Grow, Heal, Adapt, and Express Our Full Life Potential. This Is The Same Innate Wisdom That Creates An Entire Human Being From Two Cells And Causes Roots To Grow Downward and Shoots To Grow Upward No Matter How The Seed Is Planted.

In Human Beings, Innate Intelligence Is Transmitted Throughout The Body By The Nervous System.

All Healing Comes From Above-Down, Inside-Out.

Anything That Interferes With The Proper Function Of The Nervous System Distorts The Expression Of Innate Intelligence, Leading To Dis-Ease, A State Of Imbalance Within The Body.

Left Uncorrected, Subluxations Cause Breakdowns In Brain And Body Function, Leading To Incomplete Expression Of Health And Life.

All Interference To The Nervous System Comes From One Of Three Sources: Physical, Chemical, and Emotional.

Removing Nerve Interference Through Chiropractic And Maximizing Physical, Chemical, and Emotional Well-Being Through A Wellness Lifestyle Allows Us To Live To The Maximum Of Our Human Potential.

Chapter 4

Your Wellness Profile

The most important step in creating the life of your dreams is to determine your greatest opportunities for improvement. The Wellness Profile does just that. When you are finished, you will have a complete picture of your Wellness and will learn the areas that can make the biggest difference in the quality of your life. Your Wellness Profile will also help you make the best use of this guidebook.

This exercise will take time, energy and focus. However, you will find it incredibly revealing if you put your heart into it. It will be worth the effort a thousand times over.

The entire process will take about 45 minutes, so set aside enough time to complete the entire process at one time.

Step 1) Complete the Wellness Questionnaire, beginning on the next page. Write your answers in the corresponding blank on the answer sheet. Complete all the questions before scoring.

Step 2) Use the answer key to determine your scores for each question. Then add together the scores in each area of Wellness.

You may want to use a calculator for this part. Finally add these 12 scores together to determine your overall Wellness Quotient.

Step 3) Complete the Wellness Wheel with your scores from the questionnaire. Starting at 12:00 and going clockwise, place a dot at the point on the line that matches your score in that category.

Step 4) Take some time to think about your Wellness Wheel. What does it tell you about your life? What does it tell you about how you can improve your quality of life?

Step 5) Complete the exercise at the end of Chapter 5, ranking the 12 areas of Wellness.

Wellness Profile Questionnaire

Select the best answer to each of the following questions and write the letter in the corresponding blank on the answer sheet. Be totally honest and use your first "gut" feeling—this will help you achieve the best results possible.

Pain and Symptoms

1. My current (over the past week) symptom(s) and/or pain is:
   a. None at all.
   b. A minor nuisance.
   c. Somewhat bothersome.
   d. Beginning to impact how I feel and what I do.
   e. Substantially painful or restricting what I can do.
   f. Hard to take, severe pain/symptoms.
   g. Excruciating—pain/ symptoms are dominating my life.
2. My recent (past 3–6 months) symptoms have been:
   a. None at all.
   b. A minor nuisance.
   c. Somewhat bothersome.
   d. Beginning to impact how I feel and what I do.

   e. Substantially painful or restricting what I can do.
   f. Hard to take, severe pain/symptoms.
   g. Excruciating—pain/ symptoms are dominating my life.

3. In general over the past 1–10 years my symptoms have been:
   a. None at all.
   b. A minor nuisance.
   c. Somewhat bothersome.
   d. Beginning to impact how I feel and what I do.
   e. Substantially painful or restricting what I can do.
   f. Hard to take, severe pain/symptoms.
   g. Excruciating—pain/ symptoms are dominating my life.

Overall Health

4. My current health is best described as:
   a. Perfect. I have no known health conditions.
   b. Excellent. I have one or two minor conditions, and they don't really affect my life.
   c. Good. I have one or two conditions that are starting to concern me or a few minor ones.
   d. Fair. I have one or two moderate or several minor conditions somewhat affecting my life.
   e. Concerning. I am very concerned about one or more health conditions.
   f. Poor. My health condition (s) are significantly affecting my life.
   g. Failing. I have one or more severe or life-threatening illnesses.
5. My past health is best described as:
   a. Perfect. I have no known health conditions.
   b. Excellent. I have one or two minor conditions, and they don't really affect my life.

c. Good. I have one or two conditions that are starting to concern me or a few minor ones.

d. Fair. I have one or two moderate or several minor conditions somewhat affecting my life.

e. Concerning. I am very concerned about one or more health conditions.

f. Poor. My health condition (s) are significantly affecting my life.

g. Failing. I have one or more severe or life-threatening illnesses.

6. I get sick:

a. Never or almost never. B. Rarely. C. Sometimes. D. Often. E. Always.

Energy and Vitality

7. In general, the following statement best describes my energy and vitality:

a. I feel great all the time, wake up refreshed, and have plenty of energy throughout the day.

b. I feel energized most of the time, but run a little low on energy at times.

c. I have my ups and downs—some days and times are good, others aren't.

d. I frequently feel somewhat drained. I'd like to do more, but my energy doesn't allow.

e. I feel tired when I wake up or have some difficulty making through the day.

f. I rarely feel energetic. I often feel sluggish or foggy. Lack of energy is really affecting my life.

g. I can't wait to get more rest. My snooze button is my best friend.

8. Rank yourself on a scale of 1–10, 1 being little and 10 being unlimited energy/vitality.

Nutritional Wellness

9. My typical diet can best be described as:
   - a. Ideal. I focus on eating exactly the right foods nearly all the time.
   - b. Excellent. I eat a very well-balanced diet with few unhealthy snacks or desserts.
   - c. Good. I eat a relatively good diet, but don't necessarily pay much attention to specifics.
   - d. Fair. For the most part I eat well. However, I often eat foods that aren't particularly healthy.
   - e. Marginal. I have a typical American diet.
   - f. Poor. I eat foods that I like, often eat junk food/ soda, and eat few fruits and vegetables.
   - g. Harmful. I eat mainly processed foods, and rarely eat healthy foods like fruits and veggies.

10. If I add together the processed snacks, sodas and desserts I eat, I average ________ per day:
    - a. 0 b. 1 c. 2–3 d. 4–5
    - e. More than 5

11. I eat about ________ servings of fruits and vegetables per day:
    - a. 0 b. 1 c. 2–3 d. 4–5
    - e. More than 5

12. My supplement plan can best be described as:
    - a. I have a well-planned program of taking specific vitamins, minerals and other supplements.
    - b. I take some natural supplements that generally fit my needs.
    - c. I usually take my multivitamin.
    - d. I occasionally take supplements, but not on a regular basis.
    - e. I rarely if ever take nutritional supplements.

Physical Fitness

13. In general, the following statement best describes my level of fitness:
    a. I lead a highly active life and am extremely fit.
    b. I am relatively fit—far more than most.
    c. I am generally happy about how my body looks and feels and I stay quite active.
    d. I exercise regularly, but only 2–3 times per week. I would like to look and feel better.
    e. I have some activities, such as walking or golf, but am not terribly active most of the time.
    f. I get out once in a while, but I would probably have trouble getting to the 6th floor by stairs.
    g. I rarely if ever exercise, and most people would be concerned about my physical fitness.
14. I am:
    a. At or near my ideal weight.
    b. 10 lbs over my ideal weight.
    c. 20 lbs over my ideal weight.
    d. 30 lbs over my ideal weight.
    e. More than 30 lbs over my ideal weight.
15. If a viscous stray dog started chasing me, I would:
    a. Ponder whether I prefer to easily outrun him or stand there and fight him off.
    b. Probably be able to run to a safe spot.
    c. Probably be in big trouble.
    d. Definitely be in big trouble.
    e. Lay down and let him catch me so at least I wouldn't be out of breath.
16. Rate your fitness on a scale of 1 (poor) to 10 (perfect).

Emotional Health and Stress

17. The following best describes my emotions:

a. I usually listen to my emotions and make changes in my life, without much stress.
b. I get stressed-out sometimes, but generally feel great about myself.
c. I sometimes let my emotions get the best of me.
d. I frequently feel stressed-out when my life gets too crazy.
e. I don't let myself get too emotional—it's not healthy to be too emotional.
f. I am frequently anxious or depressed or have a hard time dealing with stressful situations.
g. I take medications for psychological reasons and/or have a clinical psychological condition.

18. When someone pulls out in front of me on the highway, I:
   a. Smile and wave, then laugh about it to myself.
   b. Do nothing.
   c. Wonder why they could drive that poorly.
   d. Mutter to myself what a stupid driver they are.
   e. Start yelling at them (in my own car, of course).
   f. Lay on the horn or give them an unfriendly gesture.
   g. Catch up to them so I can personally show them my displeasure at their poor driving.

19. I feel that:
   a. I am in complete control of my life.
   b. Things outside my control make my life difficult.
   c. Other people and events have prevented me from being happy and successful.
   d. My life frequently seems out of control.

20. When life gets challenging, I generally:
   a. Enjoy the challenge and become even more inspired and dedicated.
   b. Change my focus by reading, exercising, or meditating, etc..

c. Go to my friends/family/clergy for advice.
d. Complain to my friends and family members about the things that are going on.
e. Check with a doctor or psychologist to see if a prescription can help.
f. Want to be by myself to "escape".

21. Rate yourself on a scale of 1–10, 1 being totally stressed out and 10 being completely in control.

Family and Relationship

22. The following best describes my relationship with my family:
    a. I love everyone in my family unconditionally and we respect each others differences.
    b. Most days are great, but I occasionally get into conflicts with family members.
    c. My family relationships have mostly good days and a few bad days.
    d. I frequently feel stressed-out by my family.
    e. It seems that I am usually at odds with my family.
23. In my relationships with others, I:
    a. Don't necessarily agree with everyone, but get along extremely well with everyone.
    b. Get along very well with all of my friends and co-workers.
    c. Get along well with most people.
    d. Sometimes have a hard time getting along with some people.
    e. Prefer to stay away from certain people.
    f. I am frequently anxious or upset when dealing with other people.
    g. My boss and/or co-workers drive me crazy.
24. Rate your relationships on a scale of 1–10, 1 being very difficult and 10 being perfect.

Sleep Quality

25. The following best describes my current sleep patterns:
    a. I fall asleep easily and wake up refreshed and inspired nearly every day.
    b. I fall asleep easily, but sometimes it takes me a little while to get going in the morning.
    c. I sometimes have trouble falling asleep, and this affects my morning.
    d. I frequently toss and turn and have some difficulty getting restful sleep.
    e. Most nights are troublesome, and I don't usually feel refreshed when I awake.
    f. I hit the snooze (or want to) more than once on an average day, and often feel groggy.
    g. I typically feel worse in the morning than when I went to bed.

Social Wellness

26. If I were asked to speak to a group of 100 people, I would:
    a. Gladly accept and look forward to giving a great presentation.
    b. Accept, but I would be a little bit worried about how I would do.
    c. Accept, but I would be quite nervous about speaking in front of that many people.
    d. Get nervous, and maybe see if there was a way I could get out of it.
    e. Be very nervous, and probably turn down the opportunity.
27. In social situations:
    a. I feel equally at home with a friend, with a new acquaintance, or in a large group.
    b. I enjoy being around others, but occasionally feel uncomfortable with people I don't know.

c. I am comfortable with people I know, but uncomfortable around people I don't know well.

f. I usually prefer to stay home, rather than facing groups of people I don't know well.

g. I rarely socialize. Instead, I spend most of my time home alone or with family only.

28. When it comes to my social life:

a. I am as involved as I like, and do a number of fun activities with friends and acquaintances.

b. I do quite a bit socially, but sometimes wish I could have more fun.

c. I socialize some with friends, but not as much as I would hope.

d. I often wish I had more friends, and could do more things socially.

e. I often feel lonely, and really could use more people in my life.

f. For the most part, I don't like being around other people.

29. I am active in approximately ________ social/civic/church/social groups:

a. 5 or more b. 4 c. 2–3
d. 1 e. 0

Spiritual Wellness

30. I feel today's world is:

a. A wonderful gift from God, but humans need to take more responsibility for their actions.

b. A very good place with a few problems that should be addressed.

c. More good than bad.

d. Pretty scary sometimes.

e. A ticking time bomb because of many of the bad things people have done.

f. A frightening place to live.

g. Full of evil people who do terrible things.

31. People are:
    a. Exactly as they should be, but I love bringing out the best in everyone.
    b. For the most part good.
    c. Generally more good than bad.
    d. Some good, some bad.
    e. Usually out for themselves.
    f. Often out to get my money and other things.
    g. To be avoided as much as possible.
32. I attend church or a spiritual group, or do some significant form of personal spiritual ritual:
    a. Every week. b. Most weeks.
    c. Twice a month. d. Once a month.
    e. Occasionally. f. Only for weddings or other family events. g. Rarely, if ever.
33. On average, I think deeply about my higher power, or pray or meditate:
    a. Every day. b. Most days.
    c. Three times a week. d. Twice a week.
    e. Once a week. f. Only when something bad happens or I need something.
    g. Rarely, if ever.
34. On average, I read a spiritually enlightening book or religious text:
    a. Weekly. b. Monthly.
    c. A few per year. d. One or two per year.
    e. Every year or two. f. Only when someone gives me one. g. Never.

Career or Contribution Answer question 35 if you work. Answer question 36 if you are retired or do not work.

35. The following best describes how I feel about my career:
    a. I rarely feel like I'm going to work because I love what I do, and I continue to improve.
    b. I like my job, and may have the opportunity to advance.

c. My job is ok, but I feel I could do better.
d. I seem to get stressed a lot at work.
e. I really don't like my job, but don't know what else to do.
f. I really only go to work for the paycheck.
g. I can't stand my job, and would make a change immediately if I could.

Or

36. The following best describes how I feel about my current contribution to the community and world:
a. I am extremely busy doing many things to contribute.
b. I enjoy contributing and feel that my role is important.
c. I get involved sometimes, but wish I could contribute more.
d. I would like to contribute more, but don't know how.
e. I wish I had more to contribute.
f. I've pretty much accomplished everything I can, and I'm just living out my life.
g. I feel like I'm a burden on other people.

Financial Wellness

37. With regard to money and resources, I believe:
a. There is plenty of wealth in the world so it's possible for everyone to be wealthy.
b. For the most part, people can be wealthy if they do the right things.
c. There will always be a lot of wealth for some, but most people are relatively poor.
d. There's plenty of money, but I need to keep mine to be safe.
e. Money is limited. There's only so much to go around.

f. Most people are just out to get your money. I am very careful with mine.

g. Money is the root of all evil.

38. When I want something that is expensive, I *usually*:

a. Plan out how to acquire enough money to buy it, no matter what the price.

b. Decide whether it's something I really want and if it is worth the investment I'll buy it.

c. Buy it if it seems like a really good deal.

d. Buy it only if I have a coupon or if it's on sale.

e. Buy it if my credit card has enough available credit.

f. Grovel over the price or worry about the price, but usually not buy it.

g. Realize I can't afford it and move on.

39. With regard to tithing:

a. Everyone should tithe at least 10% of everything they make.

b. People should tithe, if they can afford to.

c. People should be able to keep their hard-earned money.

40. Pick one best answer:

a. I have a financial planner and have a complete plan for retirement, travel, education, etc.

b. I invest significantly in stocks/bonds/real estate etc., even if there is some risk.

c. I save for a rainy day.

d. I don't trust anyone else with my money.

e. I have no specific financial plan. I'm happy just to pay the monthly bills.

Answer Sheet

1. ________ score ________
2. ________ score +________
3. ________ score +________

=________% **Pain and Symptoms Score**

4. ________ score ________
5. ________ score +________
6. ________ score +________

=________% **Overall Health Score**

7. ________ score +________
8. ________ score +________

=________% **Energy and Vitality Score**

9. ________ score +________
10. ________ score +________
11. ________ score +________
12. ________ score +________

=________% **Diet and Nutrition Score**

13. ________ score +________
14. ________ score +________
15. ________ score +________
16. ________ score +________

=________% **Fitness Score**

17. ________ score +________
18. ________ score +________
19. ________ score +________
20. ________ score +________
21. ________ score +________

=________% **Emotional Wellness Score**

22. ________ score +________
23. ________ score +________
24. ________ score +________
=________% **Relationship Wellness**
25. ________ score +________ =________% **(Sleep Quality Score)**
26. ________ score +________
27. ________ score +________
28. ________ score +________
29. ________ score +________
=________% **Social Wellness Score**
30. ________ score +________
31. ________ score +________
32. ________ score +________
33. ________ score +________
34. ________ score +________
=________% **Spiritual Wellness Score**
35. or 36. ________ score +________% **(Career or Contribution Score)**
37. ________ score +________
38. ________ score +________
39. ________ score +________
40. ________ score +________
=________% **Financial Wellness**

Add all 12 totals together. Then divide by 12. This is your overall Wellness Quotient.

My current Wellness Quotient is ________%

Answer Key

1.	a=50	b=40	c=30	d=25	e=15	f=10	g=0	
2.	a=30	b=25	c=20	d=15	e=10	f=5	g=0	
3.	a=20	b=18	c=15	d=10	e=6	f=3	g=0	
4.	a=40	b=305	c=25	d=20	e=10	f=5	g=0	
5.	a=30	b=25	c=20	d=15	e=10	f=5	g=0	
6.	a=30	b=25	c=20	d=15	e=10	f=5	g=0	
7.	a=50	b=40	c=30	d=20	e=10	f=5	g=0	
8.	1=0	2=10	3=15	4=20	5=25	6=30	7=35	8=40
	9=45	10=50						
9.	a=40	b=30	c=25	d=20	e=10	f=5	g=0	
10.	a=20	b=15	c=10	d=5	e=0			
11.	a=0	b=5	c=10	d=15	e=20			
12.	a=20	b=15	c=10	d=5	e=0			
13.	a=30	b=25	c=20	d=15	e=10	f=.5	g=0	
14.	a=30	b=20	c=10	d=5	e=0			
15.	a=20	b=15	c=10	d=5	e=0			
16.	1=2	2=4	3=6	4=8	5=10	6=12	7=14	8=16
	9=18	10=20						
17.	a=20	b=18	c=15	d=10	e=5	f=2	g=0	
18.	a=20	b=17	c=15	d=10	e=5	f=2	g=0	
19.	a=20	b=0	c=0	d=0				
20.	a=20	b=15	c=15	d=10	e=5	f=0		
21.	1=2	2=4	3=6	4=8	5=10	6=12	7=14	8=16
	9=18	10=20						
22.	a=30	b=25	c=20	d=10	e=0			
23.	a=20	b=17	c=15	d=10	e=7	f=3	g=0	
24.	1=0	2=10	3=15	4=20	5=25	6=30	7=35	8=40
	9=45	10=50						
25.	a=100	b=80	c=60	d=40	e=20	f=20	g=0	
26.	a=20	b=15	c=10	d=5	e=0			
27.	a=30	b=25	c=15	d=5	e=0			

28. a=30	b=25	c=15	d=10	e=5	f=0		
29. a=20	b=15	c=10	d=5	e=0			
30. a=20	b=17	c=15	d=10	e=5	f=2	g=0	
31. a=20	b=17	c=15	d=10	e=5	f=2	g=0	
32. a=20	b=17	c=15	d=10	e=5	f=2	g=0	
33. a=20	b=17	c=15	d=10	e=5	f=2	g=0	
34. a=20	b=17	c=15	d=10	e=5	f=2	g=0	
35 and 36.	a=100	b=80	c=60	d=40	e=20	f=10	g=0
37. a=30	b=25	c=20	d=15	e=10	f=5	g=0	
38. a=30	b=25	c=20	d=15	e=10	f=5	g=0	
39. a=20	b=5	c=0					
40. a=20	b=15	c=10	d=5	e=0			

The Wellness Wheel

Mark a dot on each line at the corresponding score from your Wellness Questionnaire, then connect the dots. The Wellness Wheel is a picture of your life. If this was a wheel on your bicycle, how smoothly would your bike ride? The overall <u>size</u> of the wheel tells you how *full* your experience of life is. The <u>roundness</u>, or shape of the wheel tells you how *balanced* your life is. If your wheel is significantly imbalanced, you will do best to focus on improving the 1 or 2 most troublesome areas. If it is small but relatively round, you would do best by taking a more general approach to your Wellness.

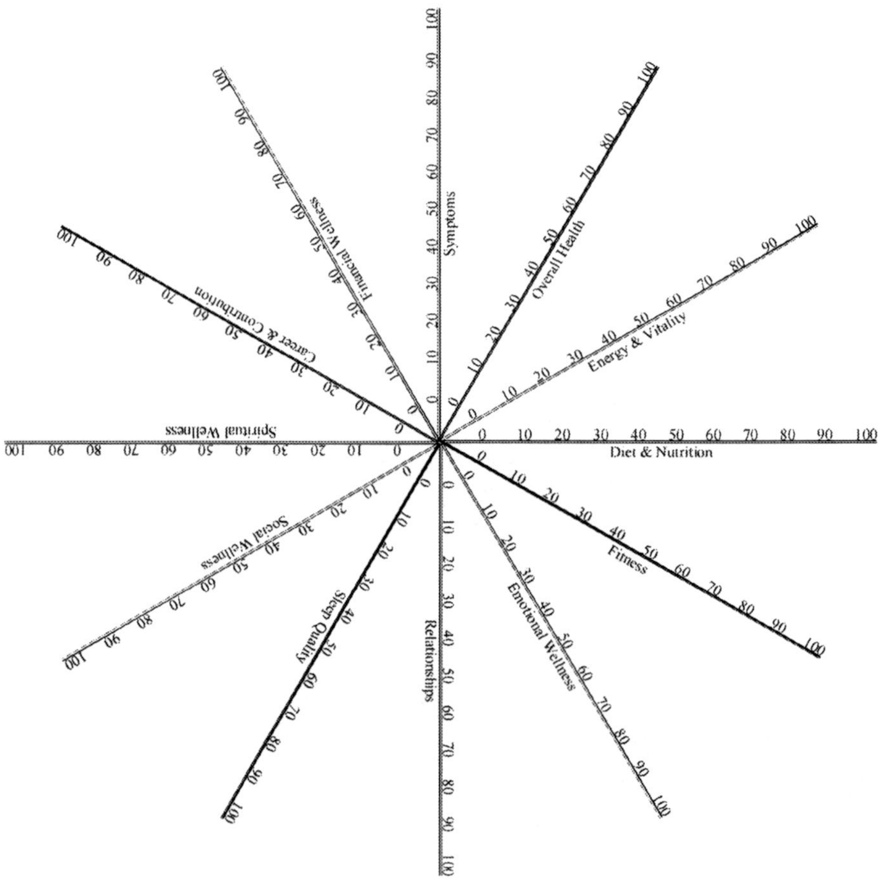

Chapter 5

Creating Your A+ Wellness Team

"To be conscious that you are ignorant of the facts is a great step to knowledge."

Benjamin Disraeli

One of the most important steps you will take in your path to Wellness is assembling your Wellness Team. You can select from a wide array of choices, including your family chiropractor, massage therapists, nutritionists, herbalists, naturopaths, homeopaths, acupuncturists, clergy and spiritual advisors, personal trainers, authors and self-improvement gurus.

This chapter will briefly explain the role each of these specialists can play. You don't need to utilize all of them—just understand that they are there for you if you choose. Some specialists, like your chiropractor, can help you in a number of areas. This would be the equivalent of a "Head Coach".

Just as these specialists have little training or expertise in severe trauma, emergencies, or life-threatening crises, most MD's have little or no training in Wellness. It makes sense to utilize medical practitioners when life or limb is in danger. However, you can only get sound Wellness advice from those who truly understand it and live it every day.

A "Wellness Specialist" is anyone who works to improve the quality of your life in a positive way. Since Wellness involves far more areas of life than physical health, there is a wide variety of people and resources to choose from. Even family members and friends can be part of your Wellness Team.

Chiropractors

Chiropractors are fully licensed doctors who fit into the Wellness model of health. As such, chiropractors are uniquely trained in a multitude of health and lifestyle areas. They often have good relationships or alliances with other Wellness professionals, such as massage therapists, acupuncturists and personal trainers.

Chiropractors can be divided into two broad categories—Medical (symptom based) and Vitalistic (Wellness based). Symptom-based chiropractors focus primarily on pain relief and musculoskeletal disorders. They take a more medical approach to care, predicating the need for care on the presence of symptoms.

Wellness-based chiropractors serve a dual role as doctor and advisor or coach. While all chiropractors see their share of symptomatic patients, the Wellness-oriented D.C. views pain relief as the *first step* of the path to Wellness. The primary focus in a Wellness-based practice is to create a life-changing experience. Clients are tracked through three phases of care; the *crisis or symptomatic phase*, the *correction phase* where health is restored, and the *Wellness phase* where the client is guided to a higher state of living. A Wellness-based chiropractor will not only address spinal and nerve function, but also other topics such as nutrition, exercise, and healthy lifestyle issues.

Proficient chiropractors provide excellent "team leaders". Chiropractors have access to other Wellness professionals, allow your body to fully express life potential, and know when it is appropriate to refer to a medical professional.

Massage Therapists

Massage therapists utilize a variety of techniques to improve soft-tissue health and function, reduce muscular and overall tension, and create a sense of Wellness.

Massage techniques range from light-touch "relaxation" massages, all the way to deep tissue techniques such as Swedish Massage and Rolfing. Make sure you discuss your objectives with your therapist and be sure that they are proficient in a technique that is congruent with these objectives. For instance, if you are under a great deal of stress and want a relaxing massage, a deep, strong technique may not serve your purposes. However, if you have significant soft tissue dysfunction or scar tissue, a light massage will fail to address the underlying problem.

Massage therapists focus on muscles and other soft tissues, much as chiropractors focus on the spine. While less direct, a good massage will stimulate your nervous system, circulation, and lymphatics. This makes massage a great companion for Chiropractic care. The combination of regular adjustments with occasional massages improves the effectiveness of both.

Acupuncturists

Acupuncture is a technique by which special needles are placed in specific places as determined by the acupuncturist. Contrary to popular belief, acupuncture is surprisingly painless. As is the case with Chiropractic, there is a large body of scientific evidence which supports the effectiveness of acupuncture. Claims that these professions are "unscientific" are simply not true—these claims are simply ignorant opinions spoken by the very people who have the most to lose as more and more people utilize these outstanding natural approaches.

Western acupuncture is provided by many American practitioners. However, this is distinctly different from traditional Eastern acupuncture. Western acupuncture typically inserts needles in various painful (Ah-Shi) points, and is designed to reduce pain and spasms (similar to the symptomatic approach of Western Medicine). This can be helpful in resolving pain and symptoms.

Eastern, or traditional acupuncture, is a unique and highly developed approach to health. Practitioners are well-trained in Eastern Philosophy. Traditional acupuncture views the body in terms of Chi, or energy. This energy flows through a number of channels, called *meridians*, supplying the body's vital life energy. In the Eastern Philosophy, health is a balance between hot (yang) energy and cool (yin) energy. Traditional acupuncturists attempt to rebalance the body's energy through a time-honored approach.

Nutritionists and Herbalists

Most chiropractors have an excellent basic understanding of nutrition and supplements. However, it is recommended that you find an additional expert in the field of nutrition and herbal healing. There are three aspects to your nutritional program:

Diet and Meal Planning

Nutritional Supplementation

Herbal Supplements

While it is always best to meet our nutritional needs through our diet, this is a very difficult task in today's world. In addition, there are a number of nutrients and supplements which are especially beneficial for certain conditions (i.e. glucosamine and chondroitin for joint health and CoQ10 for heart health) but aren't typically found in our diet. This is why it is so important to have one or more experts to help you shape your dietary and supplement program.

Personal Trainers

Personal Trainers specialize in *fitness*, an important aspect of Wellness. In the past, when we had highly physical labor and active lifestyles, most people received at least a baseline level of fitness. In today's hyper-convenience world, however, very few people get adequate exercise.

Many people envision personal trainers as the old-style, hard core, in-your-face muscle-man trainer. However, times have changed dramatically, and so have personal trainers. A good personal trainer will take the time to discuss your goals and what you hope to gain, then create a training program that fits your goals and your lifestyle.

Personal trainers don't have to create a financial hardship, either. Most gyms offer training at affordable rates. In addition, you can decide whether you simply want basic evaluation and a program setup, or if you prefer to invest more to get full-service one-on-one training. Personal trainers can be an excellent investment in your fitness and Wellness.

Naturopaths and Homeopaths

Naturopaths and homeopaths use natural remedies to address health issues. While similar in their approach, naturopathy typically uses herbs and other natural products, while homeopathy uses extremely dilute formularies to produce an adaptation within the body.

Women tend to visit naturopaths and homeopaths more frequently than men. The reason is unclear, as both genders can gain valuable healing, especially if they suffer from a health malady and prefer a natural, drug-free approach.

Naturopaths and Homeopaths can be immensely valuable, and do especially well with hormonal issues, migraines, and detoxification of harmful chemicals and waste products that frequently build up in our body.

Self-Improvement

Many of us have been taught to shun those who speak of "self-improvement." This programming comes straight out of the book of fear, which says that "If you need something to help you improve your life, you must have something wrong with you." Because of this misguided viewpoint, most people simply struggle through life, with their heads buried in the sand.

The reality is that the most "sane" and "together" people understand the vital importance of working on ourselves. There are literally hundreds of excellent books, audio programs, and seminars with a wide variety of styles. This book includes many excellent recommendations. Your chiropractor can offer even more. If you want a richer, more fulfilling life, it is imperative that you invest in yourself!

Spiritual Advisors

While not typically considered "health care," clergy and other spiritual advisors can play a vital role in Wellness. Reconnecting with your higher power can have profound affects on your experience of life. Recent research demonstrates that spiritual exercise and faith even has a significant impact on physical health.

When we think of our spirituality, we first think of clergy. However, Spiritual Advisors come in a number of other forms, including authors, lecturers and close friends. Whatever your religious or spiritual preference, seek out those who can help you on your path to greater spiritual freedom. And don't be afraid to get new perspectives—they often serve to strengthen your faith.

Financial Planners

Without a financial coach, how can you expect to attain the level of wealth, security, and financial freedom you desire? A good, holistic financial planner can help you plan, invest, and design your finances to create the resources required for your life. Trial and error has proven to be a very poor method for creating wealth.

Other Team Members

There are a number of other holistic professionals and techniques that can prove very beneficial. Microscopic blood analysis, candling, hypnosis, and others are available in many localities. Ask your chiropractor to recommend alternatives that fit your needs.

Exercise

Prioritize your needs.

According to your scores on the Wellness Questionnaire (Chapter 4), rank the 12 areas of Wellness in order of priority. Your lowest score is ranked #1.

______ Pain and physical symptoms *(Chapters 3, 6, 7, 14)*

______ Overall Health *(Chapters 1, 2, 3, 5, 6, 7, 13, 14)*

______ Energy and Vitality *(Chapters 3, 6, 7)*

______ Nutritional Wellness *(Chapter 7)*

______ Fitness *(Chapter 6)*

______ Emotional Wellness *(Chapters 8, 9, 10, 11, 12)*

______ Family and Relationships *(Chapters 8, 9, 10, 11, 13)*

______ Sleep Quality *(Ask your chiropractor)*

______ Social Wellness *(Chapters 8, 9, 11)*

______ Spiritual Wellness *(Chapter 11)*

______ Career and Contribution *(Chapters 8, 9, 10, 11, 12)*

______ Abundance and Financial Wellness *(Chapter 12)*

Now that you have determined your weaker areas, you can start to improve these areas of your life using the chapters listed.

Find Professionals to help you with your weaker areas.

Seek out the professional(s), in addition to your chiropractor, that can help you in your two weakest areas. Professional types are listed by areas they can impact most.

Pain and physical symptoms ....Massage Therapist, Acupuncturist

Overall Health ....Naturopath/Homeopath, Nutritionist, Acupuncturist

Energy and Vitality ....Personal Trainer, Nutritionist

Nutritional Wellness ....Nutritionist

Fitness ....Personal Trainer

Emotional Wellness ....Self-Improvement, Spiritual Advisors

Family and Relationships ....Self-Improvement, Spiritual Advisors

Sleep Quality ....Ask about a Chiropractic Sleep System

Social Wellness ....Self-Improvement, Spiritual Advisors

Spiritual Wellness ....Spiritual Counselors & Books

Career and Contribution ...Self-Improvement, Spiritual Advisors, Financial Planners

Abundance and Financial Wellness ....Financial Planners, Self-Improvement

PART 2

CREATING AN OUTSTANDING LIFE

Chapter 6

Living An Active Lifestyle

"The human body is the best picture of the human soul."

Ludwig Wittgenstein

When people think of exercise, they generally think of painful exercises done over and over again. This is an outdated way of thinking. We now understand that exercise doesn't need to be torture. In fact, the old notion of "no pain, no gain" is actually rather unhealthy!

In reality, there are a wide variety of options available to people of all ages and capabilities. Many of these involve a structured program, such as gyms and fitness videos. But many involve enjoyable activities such as golfing and hiking.

Don't ever let anyone convince you that they know the "best" or "only" exercise program, because exercise is as individual as your fingerprint. It is important for you to have a holistic fitness or lifestyle coach to help you match your goals with your likes and abilities to create a great program that fits into your lifestyle.

Exercise has many benefits beyond simply looking and feeling great. Obviously, activity levels have a tremendous role in cardiovascular health, obesity and diabetes. But exercise also plays a significant role in emotional health, immune function, and virtually every other aspect of health.

Designing Your Active Lifestyle

Most people have become *inactive* simply because they have no plan to *be active*! With all of life's demands and complications, things that aren't in the game plan tend not to get done. That is why this portion of the guidebook may be the most fun and exciting.

Before we begin, let's define the term ***exercise.*** Exercise is nothing more than purposely moving your body to accomplish a goal. Getting off the couch to get a glass of water isn't high on the list of recommended exercises, but *it is certainly more exercise than sitting on the couch!* Parking your car farther away from the mall entrance is more exercise yet. Taking the stairs instead of the elevator is more exercise yet. Walking to the post office is even more exercise. And how about walking the golf course instead of using a cart? Hiking in the mountains provides an even greater challenge. So does 20 minutes on the treadmill. Jogging 4 miles is even more exercise than walking 2, but running 5 is more challenging than jogging 4. Intense weight training or cardiovascular exercise provides a higher level of exercise, but running a marathon is even more strenuous.

Some of the most challenging activities people do include the ironman triathlon, adventure racing, and climbing the highest mountain peaks in the world. One of the "craziest" stories I ever heard was this guy who ran 7 marathons on 7 continents in 7 days!

When we look at exercise in these terms, we begin to see exercise as a matter of *degree*. Anyone can find a good *starting point*, create *goals*, and determine a natural *progression* to get from their current fitness to their ideal fitness. A 15 minute walk wouldn't mean much to a world class marathoner, but would be great exercise for someone who hasn't done anything in years.

Exercise

Pick one exercise or activity that you've never done (or something you haven't done in a long time). It doesn't matter what it is. Don't try to think, or plan, or analyze—just go do it!

World-Class Athletes and Young Children have two common characteristics:They are constantly moving and are extremely flexible.

When you observe the physical breakdown associated with 'aging', you will note a significant loss of those very characteristics.

Let's divide exercise into 5 general categories: Cardiovascular, Resistance Training, Core Training, Low Impact, and Lifestyle activities. All 5 are beneficial. The degree to which you should use each type depends upon your goals and fitness needs.

Cardiovascular Exercise

Walking, Jogging, Running, Biking, Treadmill, Elliptical Machine, "Aerobics", Swimming

Cardiovascular exercise is specifically designed to burn calories and increase the activity of the oxygen transport system (heart, lungs and blood vessels). Depending on the specific intensity, this type of exercise is designed to strengthen the heart, improve lung capacity and efficiency, improve blood flow, deliver more oxygen throughout the body, and burn fat.

Resistance Training

Weight Lifting, Exercise Bands, Calisthenics

Resistance Training is designed to build muscle, increase strength and fitness, improve coordination, and increase metabolism. It also improves the efficiency of the nervous system and, done properly, improves the strength and stability of the spine, pelvis, and vital joints such as the knees, shoulders and elbows.

Core Exercises

Neutral posture (abdominal "girdling"), Pelvic Tilts, Balance Exercises, Exercise Ball, Destabilizing techniques (exercise ball, wobble boards, standing on 1 leg, etc.) during resistance training.

Core Training has gained popularity because of its value in improving posture, preserving energy, and preventing injuries. Core exercises focus on strengthening and coordinating smaller muscle groups of the spine, pelvis, hips and shoulder regions. While a relatively new addition to competitive athletics and health clubs, chiropractors have been teaching core exercise for decades.

Low Impact Training

Yoga, Tai Chi, Pilates, Martial Arts, Body Centering℠

Low Impact Training has rapidly gained popularity, as it is the safest and least demanding type of exercise. Anyone of any ability, fitness level, or impairment can do many aspects of low impact training. Another great side of many low impact approaches is the integration of physical and spiritual exercise that programs like Yoga and Tai Chi provide.

Lifestyle Activities

Golf, Hiking, Biking, Mountain Climbing, Skiing, Swimming, Camping, Tennis, Surfing, Kayaking, Whitewater Rafting, Canoeing, Rock Hounding, Exploring, Kiting, etc...

Lifestyle Activities are virtually unlimited. Often underestimated, creating an active lifestyle provides fitness, excitement, enrichment and social opportunities. The happiest and most successful people in the world have usually integrated a large number of these activities into their lives.

As you can see, there is an endless supply of exercise and activities. Whatever your current fitness levels or preferences, you have a multitude of choices. The challenge is to fit exercise and physical activity into your lifestyle in a way that enriches your life, rather than as a chore.

Since there are so many options, only you or your personal trainer can select the best program and exercises for you. However, I would like to share with you the most basic (and most important) core exercise. The beauty of this exercise is that it can be used by world-class athletes—and by people suffering debilitating back pain. It doesn't even seem like "exercise". As is shown in the photos below, start in your "normal" posture. To do the exercise, simply draw in your abdomen as tightly as possible (bringing your navel in toward your spine—like a girdle or corset). Simply hold this position, and allow your shoulders to naturally roll back and your head to settle squarely between your shoulders. You should tip your head back very slightly (looking at the corner of the ceiling and wall usually works). Then hold the abdominal contraction until you feel the muscles start to quit or when you start to feel your lower back or glutes tighten. Most beginners can hold the contraction for about 15–20 seconds. Repeat this exercise over and over again. While it's best to do it standing the first few times, you can perform the "Neutral Position" exercise in any position.

The idea behind this exercise is to re-create your natural habits of proper posture and tone. So when you are in line at the grocery store, driving your car, or picking up a box, remind yourself to do this "exercise".

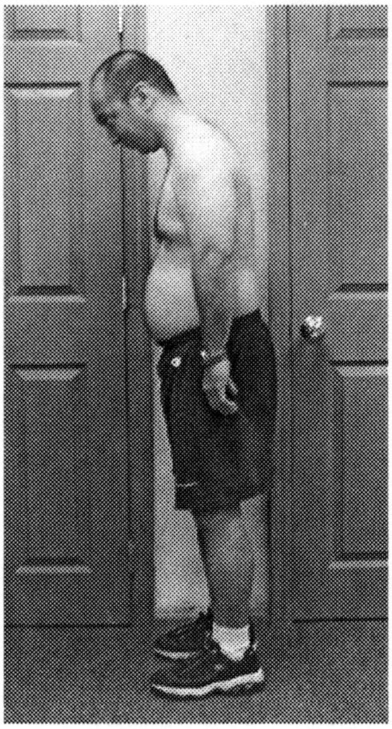

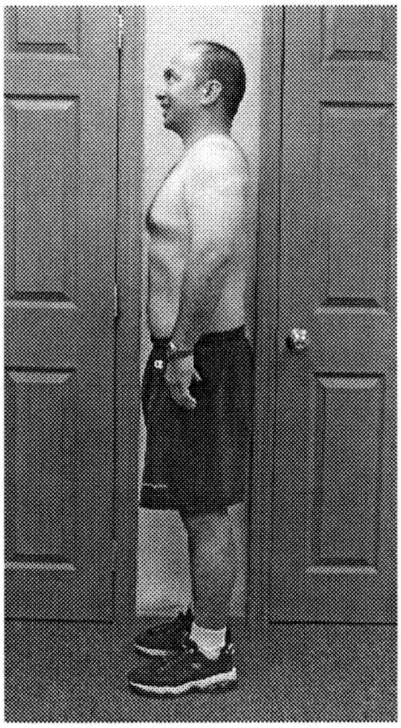

Exercise

The First Step

Pick your 5 most important goals from the list below. While most or all will have some importance to you, choose the ones best fulfill your overall health and fitness goals.

___ 1. More energy and vitality

___ 2. Activities with family and friends

___ 3. A more exciting and enjoyable life

___ 4. Healthier heart and better health

___ 5. Stress Relief

___ 6. Weight loss/ weight management

___ 7. Better posture

___ 8. Reduce neck or back pain

___ 9. Improved connection with my body

___ 10. Improved Physical Appearance

___ 11. Physical Fitness

___ 12. Reduce risk of injury

___ 13. Increase Strength

___ 14. Coordination/ Athletic Performance

___ 15. Be more able to do daily activities

___ 16. Bodybuilding

___ 17. Mental and emotional well-being

___ 18. Travel to exciting places

Now, for your top five goals (from above), use the key below and list the top exercise categories for each goal.

1. ____________________ ____________________
2. ____________________ ____________________
3. ____________________ ____________________
4. ____________________ ____________________
5. ____________________ ____________________

Key

1. Cardiovascular, Lifestyle
2. Lifestyle, Low Impact
3. Lifestyle, Low Impact
4. Cardiovascular, Low Impact
5. Low Impact, Cardiovascular
6. Cardiovascular, Resistance
7. Core
8. Core, Low Impact
9. Low Impact, Lifestyle
10. Resistance, Cardiovascular
11. Cardiovascular, Resistance
12. Core, Low Impact
13. Resistance, Core
14. Core, Resistance
15. Core, Low Impact
16. Resistance, Core
17. Low Impact, Lifestyle
18. Lifestyle

Which types of exercise appear on your list most? These are the types of exercise that will best produce the results you want. Now you can select which activities within those categories are most appealing to you. So get started right now! Never leave the scene of a decision without taking immediate action! So, **right now,** plan your hiking trip, take a walk, call your local gym, or buy a Yoga book, take whatever action is required to get the ball rolling. **Right Now!**

Exercise

Create a Comprehensive Fitness Plan

How has your first step been going? Are you doing at least 3 categories of exercise on a regular basis? If not, go back to the previous exercise and do not return to this until you have introduced at least 3 different forms of fitness into your lifestyle for a minimum of 3 months.

If you've completed the previous exercise to your satisfaction, you are now ready to develop a complete fitness plan. Including the exercise and activities you are currently doing, select at least 1 type of exercise for each category that you will be willing to do on a regular and ongoing basis.

Cardiovascular: ______________________

Resistance Training: ______________________

Core Training: ______________________

Low Impact: ______________________

Lifestyle: ______________________

Great! Now simply integrate these activities into your life. You don't have to do this all at once—it's up to you how quickly or slowly this process occurs. You should wait at least 6–12 months before moving on to the advanced level exercise below.

Exercise

Design Your Life

How do you feel after spending several months improving your physical fitness? Simply getting to this point should make you proud of yourself! So give yourself a big pat on the back. If you haven't done so already, now would be a great time to reward yourself for your efforts. So treat yourself to that new driver you've had your eye on, or that nice pair of clothes that you are now able to fit into. Or why not take a weekend to go hiking or skiing? If you've put forth the effort to get to this point, **you deserve it!** In the meantime, let's have some fun.

It is important for this exercise to be comfortable and to have no interruptions. So go to a place away from others, turn the cell phone off and lock the door.

For the next 5 minutes, visualize your ideal fitness characteristics. What do you look like? What are your measurements and clothing size? How do you feel? How much energy do you have? What activities do you partake in? Golf? A Marathon? The Ironman Triathlon?

Next, describe how your life will be once you've reached this level of fitness. How does that make you feel? Finally, make a timeline of all the changes and additions you are willing to make to develop this level of fitness. Design the life of your dreams. Read this timeline at least once a week. Have Fun!

Chapter 7

Nutrition For Life

"You Are What You Eat."

cafeteria poster slogan

There are more conflicting opinions regarding diet and nutrition than perhaps any other aspect of Wellness. Doctors saying "vitamins give you expensive urine." Scientific studies showing a profound impact of certain foods and nutrients on health. Testimonials about "miracles" happening because of a magic supplement. Unscrupulous marketers. Companies with really good products trying to help you get healthier. It's all very confusing. While our understanding changes seemingly every week, and it's certainly impossible to cover all aspects of nutrition, this chapter will attempt to provide clear guidance based upon solid science.

There is no question that our American diet is leading to millions of deaths and serious health conditions. However, with all the conflicting information, most people simply throw up their arms and adopt an "I might as well enjoy it" attitude.

This chapter will show you how to begin nourishing your body in a way that produces high amounts of energy and significantly reduces your risk for chronic illness. Common myths will be exposed. Each type of beneficial (and harmful) food type will be discussed. Guidelines based on the best available scientific research will be provided. This is a *starting point.* You should follow up with a nutritional expert, such as your chiropractor, to fine-tune your nutrition. The book *Dr. Mercola's Total Health Program* by Joseph Mercola, D.O., is an excellent in-depth reference which includes healthy recipes and sources for hard-to-find foods.* A small investment in diet and nutrition can produce amazing changes in your life.

Diet—The Cornerstone Of Good Nutrition

Nutrition is far less complicated than the media and so-called "experts" make it sound. While there are many excellent supplements on the market, nothing can replace good old-fashioned **smart eating**. It is possible, even in today's world, to eat a diet that provides most of the nutrients you need without harmful chemicals, sugars and fats. It simply comes down to making the *right choices.*

Nutritional Mythology

Myth: Cholesterol and saturated fats are the main cause of heart disease. Vegetable oils and margarines are better for your heart.

Fact: Despite the ads you saw in the 70's and 80's, consuming processed vegetable oils and oleomargarine are among the *worst* things you could possibly do to your heart. The "trans-fats" created by heat and pressure treating of soybean, safflower, corn and other oils has proven to be a much greater risk for heart disease than the butter and lard they replaced!

Lesson: Avoid <u>all</u> processed vegetable oils, shortening and margarines, except extra-virgin olive oil, flaxseed oil, coconut oil, and spreads which contain no trans-fats. Avoid all foods which contain "hydrogenated oil" or "partially hydrogenated oil".

Note: This does not mean that saturated fats are "healthy". Most sources of saturated fats are unhealthy when consumed in typical American quantities.

Myth: Lo-Fat = Healthy.

Fact: Most "lo-fat" foods contain increased levels of sugar and chemical additives. Fruits and vegetables in their natural form are your best source of healthy lo-fat nutrition.

*Joseph Mercola, D.O., *Dr. Mercola's Total Health Program.* Dr. Mercola also has an excellent website for natural health and wellness. Visit him at *mercola.com.*

Myth: Lo-Carb = Healthy.

Fact: Bad food is bad food, no matter what the "carb count". One of the most glaring examples of our cultural ignorance is the fast food industry's marketing of burgers as "lo-carb", *simply by not giving you a bun!!!* You can now choose death in a bun or death in a bowl.

Myth: Fat is bad.

Fact: Some fats *are* truly harmful, but others are extremely beneficial. In fact, world cultures that have the lowest rates of heart disease also consume the largest percentage of fats in their diet. Later in this chapter you will learn how to tell the difference between healthy fats and harmful fats.

Myth: Fat makes you fat.

Fact: Simple carbohydrates make you fatter. Consuming more calories (from any food source) than you burn will lead to fat deposition. However, because of the way the body metabolizes carbohydrates, this energy is quickly deposited into fat cells.

Myth: French Fries are a vegetable.

Fact: While potatoes are technically a vegetable, their nutritional composition is much more like a simple grain. Like other starches, potatoes are very stressful on your insulin/blood sugar system. With all the added harmful fats, french fries are the bane of any nutrition program. So why do our schools continue to feed kids french fries?

Myth: You should combine proteins, fats and carbohydrates at mealtime.

Fact: The body (especially the digestive system) has a more difficult time handling multiple types of foods at the same time. Also, certain food types are better at different times of day. Sorry, grandma, meat and potatoes is *not* a healthy combination!

Myth: You can eat what you want, as long as you take supplements.

Fact: Even with tremendous advances in the nutrition industry, supplements can *never* take the place of a healthy diet. God created a multitude of nutrients in a variety of foods. While high-quality supplements are highly recommended to fine-tune your nutrition, you simply cannot replace the nutrition found in whole foods.

Myth: The Food Pyramid was created to make us healthy.

Fact: The food pyramid was created by the government, *not* by the best nutritional researchers of the time. It was then molded by powerful political wings of various agricultural and food industry interests. It was never designed to provide the *healthiest* diet possible, but rather the *cheapest.* Since this food guide would be used to formulate school lunch programs, it was important for it to be inexpensive and practical from a food-handling standpoint. Why else would they have recommended a whopping 6–11 servings of starches, which have limited nutritional value and cause significant weight gain? The new food guide *is* better than the original pyramid, but it is still significantly flawed.

Myth: "Fruit Drinks", "Fruit Beverages", and "Fruit Juice Cocktails" count as a fruit.

Fact: Unless it's 100% pure, unsweetened fruit or vegetable juice, it's *not* juice. There is a plethora of fruit juice impersonators on your grocer's shelf. Far more impersonators than actual juices. These fake juices contain a small amount (typically 1%–40%) of fruit juice, combined with water and a host of sweeteners and additives. Other drinks and drink mixes have great fruity names, but contain no fruit at all! All of these "virtual soft drinks" should be avoided, opting instead for only "100% fruit" juices.

Myth: Artificial sweeteners and diet sodas are a good way to lose weight.

Fact: Artificial sweeteners, including saccharin (Sweet-N-Low), aspartame (Nutrasweet and Equal), and sucralose (Splenda) may be even more harmful than the sugar they replace! Saccharin has long been associated with cancer. Aspartame has been associated with altered brain function, behavioral changes, fibromyalgia-like symptoms, dizziness, and headaches, among others (and quite possibly contributed to Golf War Syndrome). While sucralose originally appeared safer than its predecessors, the truth is that very few human safety studies have been published. In animal studies, sucralose was linked to liver and kidney enlargement, and decreases in the size of the thymus gland, red blood cell counts, growth rate, and fetal body weights, as a partial list. It has also been found to contain heavy metals such as lead, and arsenic. *There is no clear evidence that these artificial sweeteners even help you reduce weight*! In fact, the preponderance of research indicates that these sweeteners actually *stimulate appetite*, leading to *more weight gain than the sugars they replaced*! The only way to eliminate the dangers caused by a "sweet-tooth" is to *eliminate your cravings for sugar through a healthy diet.* Cheating just doesn't work.

The Single Dietary Change That Can Save Your Life

Contrary to popular belief, and the USDA Food Pyramid, humans were *not* designed to consume large quantities of grains. Nor are carbohydrates found in sugars, potatoes and grains the same as the carbohydrates found in fruits and vegetables. Up until very recently in human history, we consumed predominantly fruits, vegetables, and berries along with varying amounts of wild game. Grains, such as wheat, rice, oats, rye, and barley, were introduced *as a way to provide a reliable food source to prevent starvation.* Ancient societies that consumed grains ate them in a whole, natural state. Today, over 90% of grains are highly processed—destroying whatever nutritional value they had.

Let me repeat this. Grains are *cheap*, not nutritious, especially in their usual highly processed forms. In ancient cultures (and in current impoverished societies) grains provided an insurance policy against starvation. However, if you are reading this book, starvation is probably the *last* of your concerns!

Potatoes are the most commonly consumed "vegetable" in America. Agriculturally, potatoes are considered a tuberous vegetable. But *nutritionally* (which is what we are concerned with), they behave just like a processed grain. A potato is basically starch, with a few nutrients thrown in (which are virtually all destroyed by preparation anyway). Potatoes do *not* contain the valuable nutrients and phytonutrients that make real vegetables good for you. A better option is yams or "sweet potatoes". These are somewhat less starchy, and contain far more valuable nutrients (this is what gives them their *color*).

The body processes sugars (which include "white" and "brown" sugars, as well as high-fructose corn syrup, fructose, and sucrose among others) in the same way as it processes starches from grains. The average American consumes 175 pounds of sugar per year! This equals 300,000 calories, or **800 calories per day from sugar alone!** The average American consumes 56 *gallons* of soft drinks per year, making sodas and other sweetened beverages a leading cause of sugar abuse and obesity.

There are many significant health issues related to the mass consumption of grains and sugars. We will list a few of the most common, but there are likely many more that research has yet to discover.

Obesity. Perhaps the single greatest nutritional health crisis in the United States is the epidemic of obesity. It should be no surprise that our seniors, our adults, *and especially our children*, are becoming fatter and fatter at an alarming rate. **This epidemic has not been caused by our genetics!!!** It has been caused by our **lifestyle**. Of course we live in a more "convenient" society. Of course we are less active. But the most stunning factor is the dramatic increase in the amount of simple sugars and starches we consume.

Immune System Suppression. Research has demonstrated that your immune system is significantly compromised for several hours after consuming simple carbohydrates. The best way to prevent the flu and other illnesses is to *stop destroying your immune system with sugars and starches*!

Heart Disease. OK, cholesterol haters. The party's over. The jig is up. Current research has demonstrated that the *real* dietary threat to your heart is simple carbohydrates. These sugars cause increased *inflammation* within arteries, the primary culprit in hardening of the arteries and heart disease. This is not to say that foods containing cholesterol or saturated fats are good for you (and is certainly **no** excuse to run out and grab a Big Mac). It just means that our addiction to sugar and starchy foods is even worse.

Diabetes. Most people understand the relationship between sugar and diabetes. Eating simple carbs causes a dramatic rise in blood sugar, which puts a tremendous strain on the pancreas to produce high amounts of insulin. This is also why simple carbs lead to fat deposition. Experts estimate that **one out of three children born in the year 2000 will become diabetic!** As a parent, you would never feed your child poison, right? Well think again! Those treats, snacks, fake juices, sodas, candies, desserts, cereals, white breads, and other processed foods you are using to "make your child happy" are causing irreparable harm which may eventually make your child sick—very sick—for the rest of their life!

Dr. Mercola lists the following known ill effects of excess sugar consumption in his book:

Premature aging

Cancer of the breast, ovaries, prostate, and rectum

Decreased calcium and magnesium absorption

Fatigue

Decreased energy

Reduced ability to build and repair muscle

Crohn's disease, ulcerative colitis, etc.

Osteoporosis

Yeast infections

Depression

Tooth decay and gum disease

Exercise

What steps are you willing to take to reduce the amount of sugars, starches, and grains in your diet?

____

____

____

____

____

____

____

____

The Slick Oil Industry

There's nothing like a slick-talkin' oil executive. Only the oil we're talking about here doesn't come from deep underground. It comes from a multitude of plants, mainly vegetables, seeds, and grains. You find these oils as cooking oils (soybean, corn, vegetable, canola, safflower, etc), shortenings, spreads, and in processed foods, hidden within an ingredient list that few people even read.

The entire shift to hydrogenated and partially-hydrogenated oils and spreads was based on partial and inconclusive research in the early 1950's. Several government and influential health organizations, based upon this shaky research, *proposed* that the typical diet that included saturated fats from butter, meat, and coconut oil was dangerous for the heart. Contradictory information was ignored. The soybean industry used their tremendous lobbying power to capitalize on this marketing boon. However, nobody studied the effects these alternatives would have. Then, with the political and economic support of government agencies, influential medical organizations, and virtually every medical practitioner in America, the revolution began. All because of an unproven hypothesis!

Nutritional researchers, and the few doctors who dared to disagree, were left in the dust, or even excommunicated as "charlatans" or "non-scientists". There was a powerful wave of conformity to a standard—a standard that was unstudied. This nutritional fallacy lived from the 1960's into the 1990's—precisely the amount of time needed for the full force of this disastrous policy to take effect. Instead of the expected drop in heart disease and atherosclerosis, heart disease rose dramatically, and was now affecting women in significant numbers! This is also when study after study pointed out the misguidance of the hydrogenated oil revolution.

While this is not a biochemistry book, it is important to explain, in simple terms, the skinny on fats. Let's start with a few basic definitions.

Saturated Fatty Acids: These fats, found mainly in animal fats and tropical oils, are fully "saturated" with hydrogen molecules, and have no "double bonds" between carbon atoms.

Unsaturated Fatty Acids: These fats and oils are "missing" one (monounsaturated) or more (polyunsaturated) hydrogen atoms, leading to the formation of one or more double-bonds. The best source of monounsaturated fats is extra-virgin olive oil, which is one reason why cultures that consume large quantities of olives and olive oil have dramatically lower rates of heart disease.

Omega-3 Fatty Acids: Omega-3's are found in highest levels in cold-water marine animals, and in lower levels in some plants. These are among the healthiest of all fatty acids, which is one reason why Scandinavians, American Eskimos, and other cultures who consume high amounts of cold-water fish and animals have a low rate of heart disease.

Omega-6 Fatty Acids: This is far and away the most heavily consumed group of polyunsaturated fats in the Western world, since they are the most prevalent in vegetable oils. In fact, while the balance of omega-6 to omega-3 should be roughly 1:1, the typical American diet has a ratio ranging from 20:1 to 50:1! This is a recipe for disaster.

Omega-9 Fatty Acids: Rarer than the other two, omega-9's are found in olive oil.

Trans-Fatty Acid: The most damaging fat is the man-made "trans-fat". Trans-fats are created by heat and pressure (both of which are used in processing oils). Heat and pressure cause polyunsaturated fatty acids to suddenly switch their configuration from the natural "cis" to the unnatural "trans". Trans-fats are more stable or "stiff". This is good news for shelf-life, but very bad news for your cells.

Think of a naturally occurring "cis" fat as a "soldier at ease" and a "trans" fat as a "soldier at attention". Imagine what happens to your cells and tissues when these rigid trans-fats replace the natural, flexible cis-fats. Now you can understand why trans-fats have been linked to an astronomical rise in heart disease (i.e. "hardening" of the arteries), as well as a multitude of other ill effects on our body and nervous system.

Saturated fats have long been implicated as the "evil" cause of heart disease. Let's set the record straight. In many people, overconsumption of saturated fats cause an increase in overall cholesterol, especially "bad" cholesterol. However, according to a vast body of medical research, cholesterol is only one of many biochemical risk factors for heart disease—and far from the most important! Because of their structure, saturated fats do not turn into trans-fats, even when heated. Moreover, some saturated fats, notably coconut oil, have been shown to have significant health *benefits.*

The mistake our culture has made is the explosion of processed vegetable oils. These are prevalent in hidden forms, such as eating out and in packaged foods. You likely have a tremendous buildup of omega-6 and trans fats in your tissues. For these reasons, it is highly recommended that you avoid all processed oils, shortenings, and spreads, including products that contain hydrogenated and partially-hydrogenated oils. Flaxseed oil, extra virgin olive oil, and coconut oil are three of the rare exceptions.

"But I can't bake this and this and that without those things." O.K. Don't bake this and that. It's your choice whether to change or not. It's your choice whether to continue filling your body with harmful anti-nutrients or to nourish it with foods that heal.

So what fats and oils should you use? Cook with extra-virgin olive oil or coconut oil. Use one of the new "no-trans-fat" spreads at the table. And while you should limit the amount of baked foods that you eat, use good old-fashioned butter, not processed vegetable oils or margarine when you do bake.

Because they are so rare in our modern diet, the very first supplement I recommend for everyone is omega-3 fatty acids found in cold water fish. These can be found in any health food store as EPA and DHA. For those of you who have stopped taking fish oils because of the fishy aftertaste, there are now enteric coated versions which avoid this problem. Anyone taking blood-thinning medications should not take fish oils before consulting your prescribing MD, as the fish oils can increase the anti-coagulant effects of these medications.

EPA and DHA are especially important in brain and nerve development. Therefore, **any parents who use formula for an infant <u>must</u>, <u>must</u>, <u>must</u> use formulas fortified with DHA!** In addition, omega-3's are excellent natural anti-inflammatories. Research has shown benefits for: blood pressure, triglycerides and cholesterol, nerve health, skin health and eczema, joint health, immune system, and intestinal health (IBS, colitis, Crohn's, etc.) As more research is done, I am certain that even more health benefits of omega-3's will be discovered.

Exercise

What foods in your diet contain harmful fats (including "hidden" hydrogenated fats)? Look through ingredients labels, etc.

____
____
____
____

What changes can you make to improve the quality of fats in your diet?

____
____
____
____
____

A "Steak" In Your Heart?

Another longstanding nutritional debate is the relative health or harm caused by the consumption of animal products. On one hand, the majority of Americans happily stuff their stomachs with Kentucky Fried Chicken, Whoppers, and sirloin steaks. On the other hand, a vocal minority hands out politically-motivated pamphlets on the evil dangers of meat and the "inhumane" treatment of livestock. Could anything be more polar opposite?

Let's settle the score, as much as is possible based upon the available science. As you may have guessed, the truth lies somewhere between gluttony and activism.

We, as human beings, were designed to eat both plants and animals. However, both the plants and animals we were designed to eat grew *in the wild.* The animals we ate consumed high quantities of grasses, leaves, nuts and berries (or other animals that ate those things). These animals lived an "active lifestyle" (which caused them to be lean and muscular). Most animals we now eat lead sedentary lives and eat lots of grains (which we already explained makes *us* fat—it makes them fat, too!). I remember fondly from my elementary days the cafeteria poster that stated "You Are What You Eat!" When it comes to meats, "You Are What What You Eat Ate!"

Another major concern with *all* animal products is the chemicals that come with. In the case of beef, dairy, pork, chicken and lamb, the concern is with the large quantities of antibiotics, vaccines, hormones, and other chemicals used in production. Small, but significant amounts of these chemicals travel with the meat, causing many potential ill effects in those who consume them. In the case of fish and seafood, the amounts of mercury and other heavy metals that are polluting our oceans eventually get into the fish. In addition, many species (such as salmon) are now primarily produced on farms (warm ponds where they are often fed corn—yes corn, and are often subject to runoff of pesticides from nearby fields).

There are two rules regarding the consumption of animal products.

Rule #1: Use Common Sense. Obviously, eating a double whopper is not the same as a small piece of skinless chicken breast. Prevent overindulgence. And *stop making meat the focal point of every meal!*

Rule #2: Check The *Source* of The Animal Products You Consume. Eat "certified organic grass-fed beef", "free-range chicken", "wild Alaskan salmon", wild game such as emu, ostrich and buffalo, or other hormone and chemical-free meats. Yes, these are more expensive and harder to find. But even the co-pay for your future quadruple bi-pass is much more than you will pay for *an entire lifetime* of healthy eating! These foods can often be found at your local health food store, and sometimes in your supermarket. A great resource for purchasing healthy meats is in *Dr. Mercola's Total Health Program.*

Whole Grains

As we discussed in depth, simple carbohydrates are the bane of the American diet. 90% of the grains we now consume are so highly processed as to be nutritionally empty. However, the fibers, minerals, and energy provided by **whole** grains can play a healthy role in your nutritional program. Whole grains provide a healthy energy source. The fibers are also very important for colon cleansing and function. Some grains, like oats, contain soluble fiber and are heart-healthy. Corn is the starchiest grain of all and should be limited, if not altogether avoided.

What is a "whole grain"? It is a grain that has the minimal amount of processing required. Grains are actually seeds, and have a hard fiber covering that surrounds the nutrients inside. Inside the hull are varying amounts of germ and starch. Whole grains are simply run through mills—machines that "crack" the shell (i.e. cracked wheat, rolled oats).

This is different than processed grains, which are pulverized into flour, and then subject to processing and bleaching which removes the bran and beneficial nutrients. "Enriched" flour is simply flour that has had all the original nutrition removed and then replaced by cheap, unnatural nutrients—*not* the way God created.

How do you find whole grains? It's not easy. Just because a loaf of bread is dark or says "whole wheat" doesn't mean it really is. The best way is to look at the amount of **fiber**. This is a telltale sign. If it says "whole grain", but only has 1 or 2 grams of fiber per serving—something's fishy! Even oatmeal gets confusing. While original oatmeal was very natural and whole, the "fast" and "instant" varieties cook faster because they are much more highly processed (this is why they cook faster). So if you like hot cereals, long-grain rice, etc., always select the version that takes the *longest* to cook.

The Rainbow Of Life

Fruits, vegetables, and berries (FVB's) come in all the colors of the rainbow. This should tell you something! Fruits and vegetables are far and away the most important part of any diet—and one of the most lacking in the American meal plan.

The very substances within fruits, veggies and berries that give them their greens, yellows, oranges, reds, and purples are what make them so good for us. Called *phytonutrients*, these substances have powerful cleansing, anti-oxidant, pro-immune, and heart-friendly benefits.

I won't bore you with the long list of scientifically-proven benefits (the list would be too long). So let's just leave it as follows: Your risk for heart disease and cancer is significantly determined by the amount of FVB's you consume in your life. As is the amount of energy you have on a daily basis. So is your likelihood of catching a cold or flu. Even the aging process, caused by oxidation (damage) of DNA, can be slowed by eating more FVB's. **So save yourself the chemotherapy, the bi-pass, the Kleenex, and the facelift down the road by changing your dietary priorities today!**

Vegetables

Of the three subgroups, vegetables are the most important. This is in large part because they typically provide the most fiber and are the most insulin-friendly of the three groups. While vegetables do contain significant amounts of carbohydrates, there is a common misconception that they are a "carb" in the language of modern diet plans such as Atkins and South Beach. Dr. Atkins ate *tons* of salads and other vegetables, and these are a vital part of so-called lo-carb diets.

The exception to this is America's favorite vegetable (which as we explained is not really a vegetable)—the potato. Potatoes do not fit this category. They *are* very high in simple carbs, and are very hard on the glucose transport system.

How do you introduce more veggies into your diet? Let me count the ways! You can have a side salad with many meals. Or, you can create an entrée salad (you can even top it with salmon or chicken, etc.). You can stop snacking on junk food, and start snacking on carrots, celery, broccoli, or whatever veggies you like most. You can top your sandwiches with extra lettuce. Instead of pasta (a somewhat harmful carb), you can bake spaghetti squash, and top it the same way. On a recent occasion, my wife fixed eggplant parmesan on a bed of spaghetti squash—it was as good as any entrée I've had in expensive restaurants! And get this—it had eggplant, tomato sauce, *and* spaghetti squash—3 different vegetables in one entrée. You can always do it the old-fashioned way—lightly steamed veggies as part of your meal.

Fruits

While there is no limit to the amount of vegetables you consume in a day, you do need to limit the number of fruits. This is not to say that fruits are anything but healthy. Just that many fruits contain higher amounts of simple sugars.

Some people can consume high amounts of fruits to receive the positive benefits they have to offer. Others, especially diabetics and those trying to lose weight, should consume *some* fruit, but must be careful not to go overboard. This is especially true for fruit juices and "sweet" fruits like oranges and bananas.

The great thing about fruits is that God even provided the wrapper! This makes them ideal to take to work or school, in the car on long trips—all sorts of opportunities for between meal snacks. They are also great toppers for cereal, or can be chopped up and used for dessert (instead of *desserts*)!

Berries

Berries have the highest density of phytonutrients of any food (with the exception of "superfoods" like spirulina, wheat grass and blue-green algae). This is why they are among the most colorful foods on the planet. They are often under-appreciated, as the price per pound can look relatively high on the produce shelf. But remember, these berries are toppers and snackers so a smaller amount goes a long way.

Science is just beginning to discover the incredible health benefits of berries, especially dark ones like blueberries and blackberries. Why wait? It's not like you won't enjoy them!

Superfoods

There are a number of excellent foods that contain high levels of things like antioxidants and chlorophyll. An in-depth explanation is beyond the scope of this book—you should discuss individual products with your chiropractor or health food store owner. A partial list of the best is: alfalfa, wheat grass, sprouts, spirulina, certain mushrooms, kelp, and certain algae—most notably the variety that grows in Lake Klamath.

Exercise

What fruits, vegetables, and berries do you enjoy most? Add more of these into your diet.

____

____

____

____

____

____

____

The Healthiest Choices

Here are the best choices for health-promoting foods, sorted by category.

Vegetables:

All vegetables are good for you. They are best in their fresh, natural state. Cooking or processing destroys the valuable nutrients found in veggies. The nutritional quality of vegetables, from best to worst is: Fresh organic, pesticide, herbicide, and preservative free; Fresh non-organic; Lightly prepared from fresh—(e.g. light steaming); Lightly prepared from frozen;

Moderately prepared fresh or frozen; Canned or fully cooked. Here is a short list of the many excellent vegetables you can choose from:

Broccoli, Cauliflower, Leafy Greens (the darker green the better), Cabbage, Onions, Peppers, Tomatoes, Mushrooms, Asparagus, Celery, Carrots, Peas, Green Beans, Spinach, Sprouts, Squash, Yams.

Fruits and Berries:

Olives, Avocados, Blueberries, Blackberries, Raspberries, Currants, Cherries, Melons, Red or Black Grapes, Plums, Prunes, Pears, Apples, Coconuts, Strawberries, Oranges, Bananas, Peaches, Green Grapes, Mangos, Grapefruit, Lemons, Limes, Pineapples

Proteins:

Free-range poultry, Wild Alaskan Salmon/ halibut/ etc., Buffalo, Emu, Ostrich, Wild game, Organic antibiotic-free fresh (unpasteurized) eggs (check for no cracks in shells), Organic grass-fed beef, Fresh (unpasteurized) goats or cows milk.

Grains:

100% whole grain granolas, oats, breads, cereals, etc. *with* high fiber and *without* hydrogenated oils or other harmful additives or preservatives.

Legumes (which are often considered a protein food and usually contain some fiber, but also contain significant carb levels) are a relatively nutritious food source. They include soy (the jury is still out on the benefits/risks of soy products), lentils, and the many types of "dry" beans (not green beans), among others.

Avoid all foods that contain processed grains or flour, added sugars, etc. A brief list includes most baked goods, breads, cereals, and pastas, "enriched" flour, potatoes and corn.

Oils:

Extra-virgin olive oil, Coconut oil, Flaxseed Oil, Cold-water fish or EPA/DHA supplements, other essential oils.

Use olive or coconut oil for cooking, small amounts of Brummel & Brown or other trans-fat-free spreads for topping. Keep baking to a minimum, but use butter when you do.

I also include nuts and seeds in this category (nuts are high in protein, but even higher in oils—many of which are beneficial).

Avoid *all* products that contain hydrogenated oils of any type!

Danger Foods:

Danger foods include many things you know, such as sodas, snacks, "junk foods", etc. But this list includes many things you may not consider harmful.

Chips, cookies, crackers, candy, candy bars, soft drinks, juice cocktails and other "not really juice" juice drinks, potatoes (especially french fries).

This list also includes all processed or preserved foods (frozen dinners, convenience foods, macaroni and cheese, hot dogs, chemicalized soups, etc.).

This list also includes anything that contains corn syrups, sugars, or artificial sweeteners.

It's a big list.

That's why we are *over*weight and *under*happy. And a major reason we are so unhealthy.

But as you can see, there is an even bigger list of healthy foods for you to choose from. Foods that are delicious *and* nutritious. Foods that God provided.

Exercise

Evaluate Your Diet

For the next seven days, keep a journal of everything you eat and drink. Then return to this exercise and calculate the number of servings from each group based upon your 7-day journal. You should do this during a "typical" week. Don't do this while on vacation or while your family is in town, as you probably eat differently during these times.

Food Group	Tally	Total
Example:		
Meats	IIIIIIII	8
Fruits & Vegetables (incl. juices)		
Whole Grains		
Meats (beef, pork, poultry, eggs)		
Fish		
Dairy		
Danger Foods (simple carbs and junk food)		

Next, divide the totals by 7, and enter these daily averages below.

On an average day, I eat the following servings of each food type:

____ Fruits & Vegetables, ____ Whole Grains, ____ Meats, ____ Fish, ____ Dairy, ____ Danger Foods

How does your diet compare with "ideal", which should be approximately:

5+ Fruits & Vegetables, 1–3 Whole Grains, <3 Meats, 1+ Fish, 1–3 Dairy, <2 Danger Foods

You should also drink at least 6–8 glasses of water every day.

Exercise

Make Changes

Select one Danger Food that you consume regularly. Completely eliminate this food from your diet for the next month. Replace it with one healthy food from a group you are currently lacking.

Example: "I will eliminate all soft drinks from my diet, and replace that with at least one glass of natural fruit juice per day."

Example: "I will eliminate french fries from my diet, and replace them with at least one additional green vegetable every day."

Each month, replace 1 additional danger food with a healthy food, until you have eliminated all danger foods, except occasional treats, and have all the beneficial groups covered.

Exercise

Purchase a Health-Oriented Cookbook

Page through and begin to try recipes you find enticing.

Exercise

Go Shopping

Take a leisurely shopping trip to a large health food market. Ask questions and take a leisurely trip down each aisle. Then, plan your schedule to make regular trips to this store.

Exercise

Meal Planning

At the beginning of each week or before, plan as many meals as possible, focusing on a good balance of healthy foods.

"An Apple A Day Keeps The Doctor Away!"

Chapter 8

Live Your Dreams And Fulfill Your Purpose: The Secrets Of Self-Empowerment

"Nothing happens unless first a dream."

Carl Sandburg

Without question, the most misunderstood and underutilized tool for a fulfilling life is Personal Empowerment. Why? I believe that it relates to our cultural fear of psychological and emotional issues. Too many people equate self-help to "there must be something wrong with me". This mentality comes straight from certain schools of psychology, which have told us that we are somehow "broken" and a drug is required to "fix" us. With this in mind, it's easy to understand why people are hesitant to look inside themselves or to look for assistance, whether it comes from a psychologist, book, CD, or seminar.

The vast majority of us never come close to our true potential, simply because we haven't learned how to create happiness and fulfillment within ourselves.

According to Dr. Larry Markson, founder of the Masters Circle, a world-renowned consulting firm for chiropractors, "It's All In Your Head!" He's right. In a Chiropractic office, the staff's internal thoughts, beliefs, and purpose determine the direction of the practice. In exactly the same way, ***your*** thoughts, beliefs, and purpose determine the direction of ***your entire life!*** If you are not completely satisfied with the conditions of your life, it's time to improve the conditions of your mind. That is the primary purpose of this chapter.

"Man is not the creature of circumstances; circumstances are the creatures of men."

Benjamin Disraeli

Within circles of high achievers and success masters, it is a well-known fact that our thoughts create the circumstances of our lives. According to Brian Tracy, one of the most prolific authors and lecturers in the field of human performance, our thoughts are the ***cause*** and our circumstances are the ***effect.*** Most people have it backward, believing that our circumstances cause our thoughts, feelings and actions. This is why most people go through life unhappy and unfulfilled, never becoming truly successful.

Virtually every field of human development centers on the concept that *we become what we think about most*. This includes psychology, self-improvement, and all major religions. *Successful people think about what they* ***want*** *most of the time.* What do you think unsuccessful people think about most of the time? That's right! They consistently dwell upon what they ***don't*** want.*

"Whether a man believes he can, or he believes he can't, he's right."

Henry Ford

---

*Brian Tracy, *The Power of Clarity,* CD program, Nightingale-Conant Corporation,©2001.

This is so important, let me say it again. *Whatever we think about most, good or bad, manifests in our life.* Great spiritual leaders have taught us the power of faith and belief.

"As he thinketh in his heart, so is he."

Proverbs 23:7

"We are what we think.
All that we are arises with our thoughts.
With our thoughts, we make our world."

The Buddha

So, if The Bible, The Buddha, success experts, and the world's most influencial people all agree that our lives are determined by **who we are inside** and **what we think about most**, why do the vast majority of us let the circumstances of our life dictate who we are and how we feel?

Perhaps it's because we just don't know any better. In more than 20 years of elementary, high school, college, and professional education, I received thousands of hours of training in math, science, English, history, etc. But not once in those 20+ years did anyone explain the importance of goals, of learning how to "think", or how to design my life. Most children are "told" in various ways what career they should pursue. Others simply wait until circumstances force them to earn a "living". Rarely do we ever think deeply about what we love to do or how we want to contribute before choosing a career. Why do you think so many people try so many different jobs and careers during their life, driven primarily by the simple goal of "not going broke"?

"The mass of men lead lives of quiet desperation."

Henry David Thoreau

My Story

I grew up on a well-known and reputable dairy farm. I was very successful in 4-H, FFA and other farm-related activities. There never was any question what I would study in college. The only question was whether I would return home to farm or work somewhere else within the dairy industry.

So I went off to the University of Wisconsin to study Dairy Science and Agricultural Journalism. As I approached graduation, I noticed that none of the job opportunities inspired me. So I continued my college education and received a Masters Degree in Quantitative Genetics. I did this, in large part, so that I could get a *better job* after college. But again, nothing available really tickled my fancy. I finally decided on a job in marketing and advertising in Lancaster, Pennsylvania.

My first year was great. New tasks, new opportunities to excel, and a paycheck! However, after my first year, the job became monotonous, I failed to receive the kudos I deserved from management, and I lost interest in this job. So, I decided to go to work for a competing company, move back to Wisconsin, and work individually with dairy farmers. This was it! A chance to get out of an office environment, work at the grassroots level, and receive commissions based on my performance.

This was great for the first year. Except that the farmers I was working with didn't share my interest and excitement in genetics—they just wanted cheap. And the fact that the year I started was the worst product year that the company had in over a decade, compared to an outstanding year before. So I was fighting a losing battle, and my commissions were not nearly what I had hoped for. By the end of the second year, I was finding it difficult just to get up for work every day.

Does this pattern sound familiar? It was at this lowest of low points that my life changed. One morning I woke up and realized that I just couldn't keep doing the same thing. I no longer had any desire to work in the industry I grew up in. I stayed home sick as my mind raced. No matter how much I hated what I was doing, the guilt of leaving the dairy industry was eating me up. I couldn't quit, but I couldn't keep going.

Then a bizarre flash of intuition struck me. Something inside me asked, "How would you feel if in 30 years you were doing the same thing?" Wow! In that moment, I realized that I had much more to offer the world than my current path was allowing. I immediately made a decision, called my boss, and resigned. Now mind you, I had no idea what I was going to do next. My wife and I had a small network marketing business, but nowhere near enough to pay the bills. I simply knew that something had to change, and keeping my current job wasn't acceptable.

Over the next several months, I weighed my options. I thought about psychology. My parents (bless them for this) suggested chiropractic. We struggled immensely financially, had a sickly young child, and at the time it looked like my decision was a disaster.

But at that very point in time, while at our booth at a health fair, we met a chiropractor who mentioned that our son's health problems may be related to a spinal problem effecting his nervous system. In fact, she immediately saw a problem in his neck and the way he held his head that none of the pediatricians had ever noticed. After 1 month of Chiropractic care, our "sick" son had an amazing transformation to health. It was this remarkable experience that fully convinced me to become a chiropractor.

"It is in your moments of decision that your destiny is shaped."

Anthony Robbins*

Nine years later, I consider myself incredibly blessed. I have the opportunity to help thousands of people regain their health and reinvent their lives

*Anthony Robbins, *Awaken The Giant Within,* Simon & Schuster (Fireside) ©1991.

through the power of Chiropractic and the Wellness lifestyle. And by serving others, I have the opportunity to live an abundant life. But none of this would have happened without the hardship or without the decision that allowed this path to open. And none of this would have been possible without breaking away from what I had been taught. I finally listened to that little voice inside me. This doesn't make me any different than you or anyone else—except most people are unwilling to risk *anything*, let alone *everything* to serve their highest calling.

Exercise

What hardships, disappointments and "failures" have you experienced in your life? How has each of these challenges helped direct your life in a new and better direction?

Mothers, Fathers, Teachers, and Preachers*

Most of your thoughts and beliefs are not really *your* thoughts and beliefs. You simply learned them from *others*. You learned how to act from your *mother and father*. You learned how to "think" from your *teachers*. You learned what to believe from your *preachers* (we are not talking specifically about clergy, but rather about all of your peers, the media, your culture, and other powerful influences on your belief structure). While we can gain valuable information and learn valuable lessons from the Mothers, Fathers, Teachers and Preachers (MFTP's) in our lives, we end up losing

*The concept of Mothers, Fathers, Teachers, and Preachers comes from *The Masters Guide For The 21st Century Chiropractor*, by Dr. Larry Markson, Dr. Dennis Perman, and Dr. Bob Hoffman, ©1999, 2000, 2001, The Masters Circle, Inc.

our own true identity. We spend the rest of our lives defending our *self-image*, which is not really our *self* image but a *false* image programmed into us by others.

Have you ever noticed that, just as you are on a roll, you do something that stops you just short of your goal? That's your programmed self-image telling you that "you're not good enough", "you don't deserve it", or "you always screw things up." No matter how well intended, most of the things we learned from our MFTP's, or teach our own children, derail attempts for happiness and success!

The blockbuster movie trilogy *The Matrix* creates a beautiful metaphor for the programming we receive and our struggle to find our true purpose. I highly recommend watching all three *Matrix* movies. The more times you watch each movie, the more the powerful plot that lies beneath becomes apparent. I recommend the box set, which includes an excellent discussion of the movie's plot and meaning.

"It (the Matrix) is the world that has been pulled over your eyes to blind you from the truth... that you are a slave, Neo. Like everyone else, you were born into bondage, born into a prison that you cannot smell or taste or touch. A prison for your mind.

Morpheus Speaking To Neo, In *The Matrix*

When Christianity speaks of "the flesh", Eastern religions speak of Enlightenment, Morpheus speaks of "a prison for your mind", and Psychologists speak of free will, they all describe the human battle between our *true* inner identity, purpose, and beliefs, and our *false* outside-in programming. This is the battle between our soul and our educated mind.

According to virtually all major religions and personal success experts, the secret to life is to break out of our programmed thinking to discover our higher purpose. Some call this Heaven, others call it Nirvana, and still others Self Actualization, but they are all describing the same concept! Jesus taught us that whether we are rich or poor, black or white, mighty or meek, we all have the God-given ability to change our world simply by changing our mind. We will talk more about this concept in later chapters. For now, just be aware that most of your thoughts, beliefs, and actions to this point are just programs based upon *other people's opinions*. The only thing required to transform your life is to transform **yourself**!

Exercise

What beliefs, opinions, and behaviors do you have that you simply learned from someone else? Do you even agree with all of them? Do they serve you well? If not, why do you still hold onto them?

____

____

____

____

____

____

____

____

____

____

____

The BE-DO-HAVE Principle*

One of the most important, and misunderstood, success principles is the law of BE-DO-HAVE. The BE-DO-HAVE principle is this: Your internal BEing determines how well what you DO works. What you HAVE is simply the end result of *who you are* and *what you do*.

Most people have it backward. "I'm happy because...", "I'm sad because...", "I'm poor because...", "I'm depressed because...", etc. They falsely assume that having more or different things or circumstances will change who they are and how they feel. "I'll be happy when...", "I'll act this way when..." So they spend their life looking for the "things" that will make them happy. They search for someone to give them love. They look

*Dr. Larry Markson, Dr. Dennis Perman, and Dr. Bob Hoffman, *The Masters Guide For The 21st Century Chiropractor*, ©1999, 2000, 2001, The Masters Circle, Inc.

to others for approval. They lust for money. Then they spend their money on distractions.

The worst day in the history of the world is *some*day. It seems that everyone is waiting for that someday—and then their life will change! Modern history is filled with people who "had it all" but self-destructed because they never found true success or happiness. Likewise, we've all heard many stories of personal triumph by people facing the most horrific conditions. What's the difference between these groups of people?

Successful people were successful on the *inside* long before they were successful on the *outside.* At some point they learned that by simply *changing their mind they could change their world.* Ironically, the majority of people spend their lives doing and having—trying to change the outside world. No amount of doing or having can change your being. On the other hand, the moment you change your BEing, everything you DO and what you eventually HAVE changes.

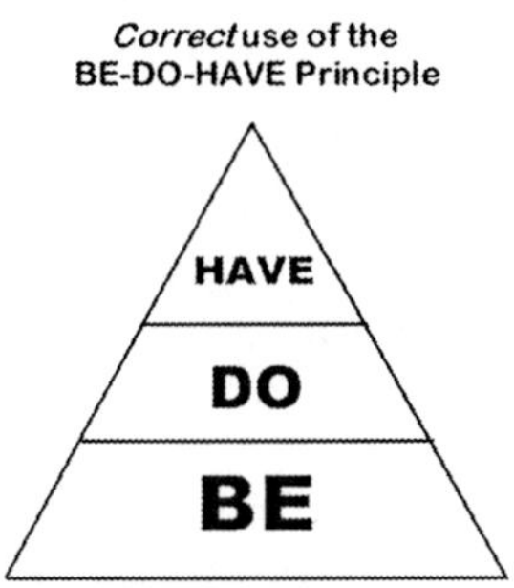

◄ The diagram on the left demonstrates that by changing who we are inside, we change the effectiveness of what we do and are rewarded by having an abundance of the things which enrich our lives.

The diagram on the right shows the common, but incorrect belief that having more things will cause us to do the "right" things and become the "right" kind of person. ►

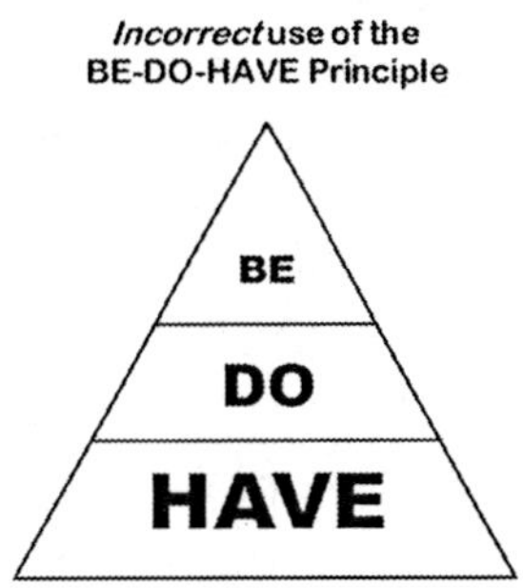

Exercise

Apply the BE-DO-HAVE Principle to something in your life. Examples: I would like to HAVE more friends, so I need to BE more friendly, cheerful, outgoing, and loving, so that I will DO the things that attract friends to me. If I want to HAVE more wealth and abundance, I need to BE more thankful for everything I already have, so that I DO the things that people do to create wealth.

If I want to HAVE ________________________________

I need to BE ________________________________

____

So that I ________________________________

____

What is Personal Empowerment?

Personal Empowerment is purposely changing your Being—creating an even better version of yourself. It is a universal law that **when you change who you are, everything else in your life changes *automatically.*** Personal Empowerment is *not* about fixing something that's broken. Nor is it vain or self-centered. Personal empowerment is about drawing out your greatest wisdom and talents to create a richer life and contributing more to the world.

Thousands of books have been written about personal empowerment. They range from the incredible insights of Anthony Robbins to the inner wisdom of Wayne Dyer to the high-powered enthusiasm of Zig Zigler. The Bible is, for many, the greatest personal empowerment book ever written.

While they vary widely in their approach, most experts agree on a few basic rules of happiness and success. This chapter is designed to introduce these basic concepts and to create a desire for you to look further into the wonderful world of self mastery.

"Life does not happen to us. It happens from us."

Mike Wickett

The ABC's of Empowerment

We will discuss the basic tools available to create the life of your dreams, including goals, affirmations, visualization, belief systems, and the power of emotions. This will form a foundation for you to build on, in any way you see fit, for the rest of your life.

Goals

A study conducted at Harvard asked one simple question of each member of the graduating class several decades ago. "Do you have written goals?" They found that only 3% of the graduating class had written goals. Years later, surviving class members were contacted. The results were astonishing. The 3% that had written goals prior to graduation had accumulated more total financial wealth than ***the entire remaining 97%!*** Of course financial wealth is not the only measure of success and happiness, but the same results would certainly apply to other areas as well.

Most people meander through life, not because they lack the talent, resources, or ability to achieve at high levels, but rather because they have no clear plan for their life. Goals are our guideposts that keep us on track and keep our life moving in whatever direction we choose.

Exercise

Set Outstanding Goals

Before starting any journey, you must first determine the best route. In other words, you must know your starting point and your destination. You can then use a map to plan your trip. A destination is nothing more than a clearly defined ***goal.*** Virtually every expert in the field of personal achievement agrees that *the most critical factor for success in any endeavor is a written list of clearly defined goals.*

We will divide goals into 6 categories: Health and Wellness Goals, Personal Growth Goals, Contribution and Spiritual Goals, Professional Goals, Prosperity Goals, and Play Goals. There are also a few rules to follow.

First, you need to be in the right state of mind. If you are feeling stressed-out or negative, get yourself into a better mindset or wait until a later time.

Second, you will need a minimum of 30 minutes without any distractions. This means no kids, no TV, no radio, and above all no phone.

Third, write your goals in the present tense, as though they have already occurred. "I am..." or "I have..." or "I do..." etc.

Finally, complete this exercise as though there were no rules and you couldn't fail. For now, do not be "realistic". In fact, be totally outrageous! So grab your favorite writing utensil and plenty of paper and lets get started.

If there were no rules and you couldn't fail, what would your health and wellness be like? What weight would you be at? How often would you work out? Describe your overall health. What outdoor activities do you partake in? Would you take lots of medications... or lots of supplements? Etc...

Health and Wellness Goals:

___

___

___

Do the same for Personal Growth goals. What are you like as your ideal self? What books would you like to read? What seminars would you like to attend? Who would you like to meet? Describe your ideal relationship with your spouse, your children, parents, friends and co-workers. Etc...

Personal Development Goals:

Contribution and Spiritual Goals. How would you like to contribute to others? What mark would you like to leave on the world? What will your epitaph say? How would you like to improve your relationship with your higher power? How much money would you like to donate where? Would you like to volunteer or take up a cause? Etc...

Contribution and Spiritual Goals:

What would you like to accomplish Professionally? Would you like to advance in your current career, change careers, start your own business? What further education will you need?

Career Goals:

How much income would you like per year? How much wealth will you acquire? How will you use this wealth? Building your dream home? Traveling? Paying for your children's college education? Leaving it to your children, grandchildren or church?

Wealth and Abundance Goals:

Play Goals. You've done the tough work. Now it's time to really expand your mind and create an incredible list of play goals. There is no reason to be ashamed about wanting nice things for yourself and your family. Select things that will really add juice to your life. Do you want a new boat? A new car? A European Vacation?

Play Goals:

Now that you have written all your goals, provide a time frame for each goal. Next to each goal, write whether it is a 1 year (short-term), 5 year (medium-term), or 10 year or longer (long-term) goal.

After you have time stamped your goals, review your lists. From each category, select your top goal. If a goal doesn't absolutely get your juices flowing, it's not compelling enough.

Rewrite each of these 6 goals *in vivid detail.* Make sure you have at least 2 short term goals, at least 2 medium goals, and at least 1 big, extraordinary long-term goal. These should be the most important, the most compelling, and the most rewarding of all your goals. This is the "working model" for your life. **Review these goals on a daily basis.**

#1 Health and Wellness Goal:

#1 Personal Development Goal:

#1 Contribution and Spiritual Goal:

#1 Career Goal:

#1 Wealth and Abundance Goal:

#1 Play Goal:

Purpose

Your purpose is simply your ultimate lifetime goal. It is the fuel which drives your passion. People who live On Purpose live incredibly rich and exciting lives, find it easy to make decisions and stick to them, live with a higher sense of love, and contribute greatly to the world. We call them Leaders.

"Nothing splendid has ever been achieved except by those who dared believe that something inside of them was superior to circumstance."

Bruce Barton

What is your Purpose? What is the ultimate way that you wish to contribute to the world? Take some time (right now!) to think this through. Your purpose should be clear, concise and to the point (one or two sentences). This purpose will be the driving force for your thoughts, actions and decisions, so be clear to let your intuition, not your Mothers, Fathers, Teachers, or Preachers determine your destiny.

Exercise

My Purpose

____

____

____

____

____

____

____

____

____

Affirmations

It is estimated that our internal dialogue consists of up to 60,000 words per day. Unfortunately, the vast majority of our internal chatter is negative. In fact, if your best friend talked to you the way most of us talk to ourselves, you would leave that friend immediately!

Where does all this negative self-talk come from? Again, it's our Mothers, Fathers, Teachers and Preachers telling us that we can't live up to the expectations *we* think *they* have for us. Ironically, we tend to think that others have higher rules and expectations for us than they actually do.

Do you ever have thoughts like, "I can't do that," "I'm just not good at that," "I can't afford that," "That's just not me," "I don't deserve that," "Why do I always screw up?" or "I'm so clumsy!"? Of course you do. We all do. The problem with these statements is that over time they tend to become generalized. Something as minor as spilling the milk turns into "I'm so clumsy" which turns into "I make a mess out of everything". A simple mistake at work becomes "I'm terrible at this job" which becomes "I can't do anything right" which becomes "I'm a failure".

It is virtually impossible for us to stop talking to ourselves. The only way stop negative thoughts is to *replace them with positive thoughts.* The human mind can only ponder one thought at a time, so when you fill it with good thoughts and positive affirmations, there's simply no room left for negative self-talk. Some people view the idea of positive thinking as Pollyanna or "looking through rose-colored glasses", but this is totally untrue. Here's the question: If you can choose between positive, healthy thoughts or negative, destructive thoughts, which would you choose? Which do you think lead to a more rewarding and fulfilling life?

Affirmations are positive statements about ourselves that we repeat over and over again. You don't even have to "believe" an affirmation at first. Many of the thoughts you have about yourself are completely untrue, but you think they are real, simply because you have heard them repeated them enough times. The same thing holds true for affirmations. Even if an affirmation isn't totally true right now, if you repeat it with emotion enough times, your mind will believe it. And once your mind believes a positive affirmation, it will *automatically* begin to take action based upon that affirmation.

Let's say, for example, that you tend to procrastinate. So you buy books on procrastination, try to learn how to not be a procrastinator, and feel guilty about your procrastinating behavior. Guess what? At the end of the day… you're still a procrastinator! Why? Good intentions aside, you've actually *strengthened* the belief that you are a procrastinator! Instead, create a positive affirmation such as "I am action-oriented." or "I love getting things done **right now**!" and then repeat this affirmation over and over again. Before long, you will have ***no choice*** but to start getting things done on time!

Exercise

Your Daily Affirmations*

Create a list of your daily affirmations. These should be congruent with your goals and purpose. Think about what characteristics you would need to have to accomplish your goals.

Affirmation Guidelines

Affirmations must be in the **first person.** ("I am…")

Affirmations must be in the **positive** ("I am a non-smoker" *not* "I am not a smoker")

Affirmations must be in the **present tense** ("I eat foods that nourish me." *not* "I will go on a diet next month.")

Affirmations must be **read out loud** with emotion and enthusiasm. This opens the "trap door" between conscious and subconscious.

Affirmations are best done in the early morning, before you become preoccupied with negative thoughts and in the evening, just before bed, so your subconscious can dwell on positive thoughts during sleep.

Carry a crib note of your affirmations with you wherever you go, so if you begin to feel down, negative, or stressed, you can immediately call upon your affirmations to get back in the game.

*Adapted from Dr. Larry Markson, Dr. Dennis Perman, and Dr. Bob Hoffman, *The Masters Guide For The 21st Century Chiropractor,* ©1999, 2000, 2001, The Masters Circle, Inc.

So, create your list of Affirmations, and read them out loud at least once every day!

A Few Examples of Affirmations:

"I like myself!"

"I can accomplish anything I put my mind to!"

"I am action-oriented!"

"I am incredibly successful."

"I am a great... mother/father/spouse/thinker/leader/business owner/etc.!"

"I am grateful for all of the abundance God has provided me!"

"I am a master!"

"I am a visionary!"

"I love saving money and am creating wealth and security for my family!"

"I am incredibly healthy!"

"I deserve to be healthy/wealthy/happy!"

"I am a very loving person!"

My Affirmations

I am…

Visualization

Once you have set your goals, determined what characteristics you will need to achieve these goals and created a list of affirmations to bring out those characteristics, it's time to get your mind focused on what it is you really want. Visualization is creating a picture of your goal, in vivid detail, as if it has already occurred. Some call this "daydreaming". That's ok. The list of history's biggest daydreamers includes Thomas Edison, Albert Einstein, Ben Franklin, Mozart, Picasso, Alexander Graham Bell, and the Wright Brothers! The word daydreaming implies a lack of focus, but visualization actually clears out all the mental clutter and puts your entire focus on the goal at hand.

"The human mind cannot distinguish between an actual event and something imagined vividly and in great detail."

Maxwell Maltz, M.D., Developer Of Psychocybernetics

In a famous experiment by Maxwell Maltz, one group actually practiced shooting free throws over and over again during the course of the study. Another group simply visualized (imagined) shooting and making free throws for a given time period. **At the end of the study, those who only *visualized* the free throws were able to make free throws at almost exactly the same percentage as those who had actually practiced physically!** I once listened to an ex-POW from Vietnam who spent his time in his underground cell visualizing round after round of golf. When he was finally freed and came home, he discovered that his golf game had improved so dramatically that he actually joined the pro tour for a short time! How's that for the power of intense focus and visualization?

"Imagination is more important than knowledge."

Albert Einstein

At the beginning of this chapter we talked about how our thoughts create our life and how people manifest what they think about most. Visualization is the tool which allows our thoughts, our vision, to manifest in our lives.

Wealthy people think about investing; Poor people think about being broke.

Happy people think about all the good things in their life; Unhappy folks dwell on what they're missing.

Successful people focus on their successes; Failures dwell on their "failures".

Great orators think about moving their audience with passion; Bumblers worry about forgetting their lines.

Winners think about winning; Losers think about losing.

Exercise

Visualization

Select one of your primary goals. After reading these instructions, close your eyes and imagine the goal as if it were already accomplished. Continue to add detail. What does it look like? What does it sound like? What does it feel like? Continue to add visual and sound details until you feel a sense of joy, bliss and pride for having accomplished this goal. Then, at the peak of this experience, think about how it makes you feel in this moment.

Do this exercise often. Every great human accomplishment is the result of vision.

Belief Systems

Ultimately, our decisions and actions are all expressions of our underlying beliefs. No matter how hard we try or what skills we develop, our minds will not allow us to go against our beliefs. If you are achieving great things in your career, but have a hidden belief that you are a failure or don't deserve to earn more money, at some point your mind will cause you to sabotage your advancement.

There is a true story about a young man who went to Harvard. Halfway through his first semester, he was called into the Dean's Office because he was failing every single class. When the Dean asked him why he was having so much trouble, the young man explained. "When I got my acceptance letter, I was surprised that you accepted me because my IQ was below average. It is very difficult for someone of below average intelligence to do well at such a prestigious university." The baffled Dean asked him what he meant. The student replied, "In my letter it stated that I scored a 99 on my IQ test."

"Young man," said the Dean, "That isn't an IQ score, it's a *percentile.* You scored higher than 99% of all college applicants!" Not only was he one of the "smartest" students in his class, he was one of the smartest college students in the entire country! Once he realized this, his grades rose immediately and he became a straight A student.* Never underestimate the power of belief!

"Life is like a box of chocolates."

Forrest Gump

Most people think our beliefs are "hard wired" and unchangeable. But you can change any belief that you want to. In fact, most of our beliefs were acquired from others—they aren't even our own beliefs! As you will learn in the exercise, you can purposely select which beliefs empower you, and which beliefs disempower or limit you. You can then strengthen your

*Brian Tracy, *The Power of Clarity,* CD program, Nightingale-Conant Corporation ©2001.

empowering beliefs and weaken, destroy or completely redefine your limiting beliefs.

Exercise

Create an Empowering Belief System*

Take some time to write down as many beliefs as you have. A belief can range from a simple opinion about something to a deep conviction. At this point, don't try to make your beliefs right or wrong, "good" or "bad". Simply write down the first things that come to mind.

Global Beliefs:

Beliefs about people in general

People are...____

People are...____

Beliefs about the world

The world is...______________________________________

The world is...______________________________________

Beliefs about life

Life is...____

Life is a...____

Beliefs about yourself

I am...____

I am a...____

*Adapted from Dr. Larry Markson, Dr. Dennis Perman, and Dr. Bob Hoffman, *The Masters Guide For The 21st Century Chiropractor,* ©1999, 2000, 2001, The Masters Circle, Inc.

Identity Beliefs:

Beliefs about yourself as a person

Beliefs about yourself in the workplace/career

Beliefs about yourself in relationships with spouse, parents, children

Beliefs about yourself spiritually

Contextual Beliefs:

Beliefs about your family and background

Beliefs about money, wealth and prosperity

Beliefs about service

Beliefs about contribution and making the world a better place

Limiting Beliefs:

While you may find you have limiting beliefs in other categories, the following concepts are common areas for limiting our lives.

Beliefs about poverty

Fear of confrontation or rejection

Fear of failure

Fear of success

Fear of inadequacy

Time and energy management

Now that you have written down a number of beliefs, evaluate each one to determine whether they empower you to achieve your goals and purpose or if they limit you in any way from what you want. Make a separate list for your Empowering and Limiting Beliefs.

Empowering Beliefs:

Limiting Beliefs:

Finally, begin to *weaken* your limiting beliefs and *strengthen* those beliefs which empower you. Ask "What do I want to believe?" and "What would I need to believe in order to reach my goals?" There are a number of advanced techniques to change belief systems. Here are a few.

Challenging Limiting Beliefs:

Prove the belief wrong. Think of examples that differ from this belief.

Question the belief. How do you know? Is it even *your* belief?

Provide leverage. What is it costing you to have this belief?

Reframe the belief. Does it only apply to certain situations?

Determine what you need to make the belief untrue. Education? Skill? Confidence?

Creating or Strengthening Empowering Beliefs:

Affirm the belief through positive self-talk/ affirmations.

Make a list of everything you can find to validate the belief.

Hold yourself to a higher standard.

Supercharging Your Life With Emotions

It seems that most people are in an eternal battle with their emotions. This is unfortunate, as it is our emotions that paint our uniquely human portrait. We are taught that our emotions are "bad", something to fear, as though they were given to us by the devil himself.

Chapter 11 of Anthony Robbins' Bestseller *Awaken The Giant Within* deals very eloquently with emotions.* Many of those concepts are used in the more abbreviated discussion provided here.

People deal with emotions in three basic ways:

Denial. Through denial, we simply ignore our emotions, hide them from others, and pretend that they don't matter. Or we altogether avoid experiences that may produce our less comfortable emotions. This actually creates more emotional turmoil as we live our lives running and hiding.

Embellishment. Some people use the exact opposite approach. These people take a "woe is me" point of view and decide to fully indulge in their painful emotions. They are quick to tell others how terrible they have it and even compete with others, trying to convince them that they have it worse. They sometimes even rely on drugs (prescription or illicit) to help them deal with their "broken" emotional health.

Awareness and Understanding. In order to fully experience life, you *must* let your emotions work *for* you, not against you. You can't run. You can't hide. But you also can't let them run your life. By learning to listen to your emotions and using them to your advantage, you can vastly improve the fabric of your life. This means you allow yourself to feel painful emotions, listen to what those emotions are trying to tell you, then take action to change the situation. It also means giving yourself permission to fully engage in empowering emotions.

*Anthony Robbins, *Awaken The Giant Within,* Simon & Schuster (Fireside) ©1991.

The first step to properly deal with your emotions is to take inventory of both "positive" emotions, which Anthony Robbins calls **Power Emotions**, and uncomfortable emotions, which I call **Wake-Up Calls**.

There are 2 things you will learn in the exercise. First, you will learn the messages Wake-Up Calls are sending you, and how to *take action* in response. Second, you will learn how to feel your most valuable Power Emotions whenever you want.

Exercise

Making Your Emotions Work *For* You

Create a full list of all the emotions you feel on a regular basis, putting each emotion on the appropriate chart below.

Some Examples of Power Emotions

Love, Happiness, Gratitude, Excitement, Adventure, Passion, Determination, Faith, Flexibility, Contribution, Vitality, Fun, Joy, Confidence, Leadership, Courage, Success, Commitment, Creativity, Cheerfulness

Some Examples of Wake-Up Calls

Discomfort, Boredom, Fatigue, Embarrassment, Fear, Worry, Anxiety, Hurt, Anger, Frustration, Disappointment, Defeat, Guilt, Shame, Regret, Grief, Unworthiness, Inadequacy, Overwhelm, Depression, Helplessness, Loneliness

Power Emotions

____

____

____

____

____

____

____

____

____

____

Wake-Up Calls

Now, look at your list of Power Emotions. Which one is the most important to you (makes you feel the most passionate when you feel it)? The second most important? Reorganize your list to include your Top 10 Power Emotions in order of importance. For each one, name something that you do or think about that causes you to feel that emotion. Example: "When I'm happy, I smile." or "I feel loving whenever I think of my wonderful children." Now you have an *anchor*, or tool, **so you can feel any of your Power Emotions *whenever you choose to!*** So create an anchor for each of your Power Emotions to call upon whenever you need to or want to.

Do the same with your Wake-up Call list, except describe what each of these emotions is telling you. Then *take positive action* based upon what the uncomfortable emotion is telling you. There is an excellent in-depth description of this in *Awaken The Giant Within.*

Less intense emotions like discomfort, embarrassment and boredom tell you that something isn't quite perfect. What is it that is causing your discomfort? Is it worth feeling uncomfortable? If so, fine-tune your approach.

Emotions such as fear, worry and anxiety are wake-up calls to "Be Prepared". Perhaps you need to gain more information. Perhaps you need to practice or sharpen your skills. Or maybe you simply need to have faith.

Emotions of hurt and anger mean that someone has broken one of your rules or one of your strongly held beliefs. The solution to these emotions is to clearly explain to the other person that what they did made you feel a certain way. Remember, it's *your* rule or belief, not theirs! So don't make them wrong. You may even find that what they did was completely unintentional.

Frustration means that you know you can do better. This is an exciting wake-up call! Get curious about this emotion. Perhaps you are simply looking at things wrong or are being impatient. Or perhaps it's time for you to make a change in your life.

Disappointment and defeat are more difficult. These emotions mean that something you really wanted is not likely to happen. But remember, sometimes disappointments are exactly what we need to find what we really want. So immediately change your focus and goals to something even more compelling.

Guilt, shame, and regret are emotions designed to tell you that you broke one of your own rules. But rather than wallow in these emotions, use them to hold yourself to a higher standard.

Unworthiness and inadequacy signal that you don't feel like you are contributing enough. There are two things you must do. First, reconsider your role on earth. In what ways have you contributed throughout your life? In what new and exciting ways can you contribute in the future?

Depression, helplessness and overwhelm are telling you that you have bit off more than you can chew. So as soon as you feel these emotions, you need to decide what is really most important. Then focus on that. One thing at a time. Deal with the less important things at a later time.

Loneliness is the most disempowering emotion of all. It means that you don't feel connected. If you feel emotions of loneliness, it's time to reach out to others—friends, family, or even perfect strangers. And remember, you can never be truly alone.

Top Ten Power Emotions	**How I can create this state any time I choose**
1.	
2.	
3.	
4.	
5.	
6.	
7.	
8.	
9.	
10.	

Top Ten Wake-Up Calls	**The message this Wake-Up Call is sending me**
1.	
2.	
3.	
4.	
5.	
6.	
7.	
8.	
9.	
10.	

So your mission is clear. Decide which Power Emotions are most important to you and your purpose. Learn how to feel these emotions all the time. Determine which Wake-Up Calls you are experiencing most often and ask what action they are telling you to take. So get to work and watch the quality of your emotional life skyrocket!

"We know too much and feel too little. At least we feel too little of those creative emotions from which a good life springs."

Bertrand Russell

Exercise

Your Daily Success Ritual

Devote a minimum of 15 minutes every day to goals, affirmations, visualization, prayer, meditation, exercise, and other personal empowerment activities. Make this as much a part of your daily routine as bathing, eating, and brushing your teeth. Ideally, you will spend 1 hour every day on this exercise.

Activities I Can Use In My Daily Success Ritual

1. ______________________________

2. ______________________________

3. ______________________________

4. ______________________________

5. ______________________________

6. ______________________________

7. ______________________________

8. ______________________________

Exercise

Learn From The Experts

If you haven't already done so, purchase a book or CD set from the reference list. Read or listen, and **do what they teach.**

Create Your Success Library

Purchase a minimum of 10 books or audio programs to begin your success library. These can come from the references list or from other recommendations. As you continue to grow, continue to add to your success library.

Chapter 9

The Magic Of The Enneagram: Your Personality Type

"You Will Know The Truth,
And The Truth Will Make You Free."

Jesus of Nazareth

Understanding Your Personality Type

Why do two people, given the same basic life situation, react completely differently? How can one read a book or attend a particular seminar and create dramatic changes in their life, while the other, reading the same book and attending the same seminar accomplishes no change at all? A major part of the answer to these questions is *personality*. Your personality is as unique as your fingerprint. You filter everything you perceive and learn through your distinct personality. The tragedy is that few of us ever learn why we act and react the way we do.

There is a fascinating field of personality study, which began about 5,000 years ago, that has been revised and revisited during the 20th century. Called the Enneagram, it is a system which describes nine distinct personality types, and can be used as a tool for growth and enlightenment, as well as a way to better understand others.

A brief description of each of the nine types is included here. However, to find your type and really learn about yourself and others, we recommend that you read the books that provide a more complete explanation, such as *The Wisdom Of The Enneagram*, by Don Richard Riso and Russ Hudson, *Discovering Your Personality Type*, by Don Richard Riso, and *Enneagram Made Easy*, by Baron and Wagele.

Type 1: Logical and self-controlled, responsible and dedicated. Judge people and situations based upon right and wrong. Tend not to be outwardly emotional. Can be perfectionistic.

Type 2: Very responsible and dedicated to others, including work, friends, and family members. Enthusiast helpers. May sacrifice themselves to support other people, missions, or activities.

Type 3: Very independent and assertive. Extremely goal and achievement oriented. May sometimes sacrifice themselves and others to achieve their goals. Highly image-driven.

Type 4: More melancholy, withdrawn and individualistic than other types. Very active internal imagination and creativity, can be dark and eerie. Want to be acknowledged by others, but also view themselves as different and special. Often uniquely creative, musical, or artistic.

Type 5: Withdrawn and logical. Often spend time "inside their own head". Typically very ingenious and intelligent. Less emotional than other types, except when their expertise is questioned. Usually more intellectual than physical or athletic.

Type 6: Very responsible and dedicated, but fearful of change. Have strong feelings about things, but may not speak out for fear of being wrong. Don't want to be controlled, but often have difficulty making decisions for themselves. Often expect the worst and evaluate things based upon risk or "What-if".

Type 7: Very adventurous risk-takers. Like to try new things, are uncomfortable with sameness. Have excellent imaginations and creativity, but often get bored with details. Great starters, but leave many unfinished projects. Love to have fun and are often the life of the party.

Type 8: Very strong and independent. They "wear the pants in the family". They are powerful, but potentially abrasive leaders. May have a hard time understanding the feelings of others or see feelings as weakness. Hard workers, but tend to under-appreciate the efforts and opinions of others.

Type 9: The most quiet and peaceful type. They avoid conflict whenever possible, and tend to take the middle ground. Kind and gentle, but can lack assertiveness and may avoid important issues. Often provide a quiet, but positive outlook and presence.

Remember that none of the types are "good" or "bad". So start with the one that seems to fit you the best. If you had difficulty finding your type, read more about each possible type. If the description of a type really sounds like you, it probably is. But again, you should do further testing and research to know for sure. If your chiropractor is familiar with the Enneagram, they will likely be able to help.

"He who cannot change the very fabric of his thought will never be able to change reality."

Anwar Sadat

The Nine Personality Types Of The Enneagram

Type 1: The Perfectionist

A.K.A. The Reformer, The Teacher, The Activist, The Crusader, The Moralist, The Organizer

The primary need of a One is to live life the right way.

The primary thoughts of a One are "How could you do that?" and "This is just the way it's supposed to be done."

At their best, Ones are idealistic, rational, self-disciplined, orderly, ethical, fair, and honest, but they can also be overly strict and serious, critical, judgmental, controlling, jealous, and intolerant. They look down on people who "break the rules," but are even more critical of themselves for their perceived imperfections.

Ones grow by allowing themselves to be more spontaneous, being more open-minded and less opinionated, learning about views that are different than their own, and being easier on themselves and others.

Ones must be careful to avoid becoming rigid and inflexible, self-righteous and overly judgmental, or being too hard on themselves. These are characteristic signs of stress for a One.

Famous Ones include: Ghandi, Martha Stewart, Al Gore, Hillary Clinton, John Paul II

Type 2: The Helper

A.K.A. The Caretaker, The Doting Mother, The Pleaser, The Special Friend, The Enabler, The Lover, The Rescuer

The primary need of a Two is to be loved and valued.

The primary thought of a Two is "Let me help."

At their best, Twos are altruistic, caring, generous, demonstrative, loving, helpful, considerate, and compassionate, but they can also become martyrs, become manipulative, possessive and hysterical. Twos often care for others at their own expense, but in reality their desire to help others stems from their own need to be needed. They are the people who always show up to the company picnic with brownies when everyone else forgot, and often have a life full of strays—stray people, stray family members, and often stray animals.

Twos grow by focusing on their own needs, especially their emotional needs. Learning self-expression through music, art, and writing or journaling can be very healthy for a Two.

Twos must be careful to avoid manipulating and coercing others, obsessive love or attachment, acting out, feeling "entitled", and often somatization (physical symptoms caused by emotional issues).

Famous Twos include: Mother Theresa, Ann Landers, Eleanor Roosevelt, Arsenio Hall, John Denver

Type 3: The Achiever

A.K.A. The Motivator, The Communicator, The Role Model, The Status Seeker

The primary need of a Three is to achieve success and to be important.

The primary thought of a Three is "I need to be the best."

At their best, Threes are ambitious, confident, driven, energetic, and self-assured, but they can also be narcissistic, vain, superficial, deceptive, and overly competitive. Threes are achievement and status oriented. They frequently excel at whatever they do, but often at the expense of friendships and their own welfare.

Threes grow by shifting their focus to goals that are bigger than themselves (serving the greater good). They also grow through teamwork, not for personal acclaim, but simply to achieve a common goal. They can achieve surprising satisfaction through selfless acts.

Threes must be careful to avoid workaholism, projecting a false image, inner emptiness, unrealistic expectations of success, episodes of rage or hostility, or taking advantage of others.

Famous Threes include: Bill Clinton, Elvis, John Travolta, Oprah Winfrey, Barbara Streisand, Michael Jordan

Type 4: The Tragic Victim

A.K.A. The Artist, The Individualist, The Romantic

The primary need of a Four is to be understood.

The primary thoughts of a Four are "What's the meaning of life?" "I'm unique." and "Why me?"

At their best, Fours are creative, introspective, intuitive, and expressive, but they can also be melancholy, depressed, withdrawn, self-conscious, moody, and self-absorbed. They can create incredible expressions of their inner thoughts and feelings, often through the arts or by being incredibly romantic—if they can only keep from self-destructing through depression and moodiness.

Fours grow by becoming engaged. By breaking out of their own internal scenarios to create meaningful action. This is why Fours so often suffer through long periods of unhappiness, but then become incredibly inspired when they begin to apply themselves through work, art, music, writing, or friendships.

Fours must be careful to avoid a sense of alienation, emotional volatility, outbursts of rage, hostility and hatred, chronic depression, hopelessness, and obsessions with death, morbidity, and self-hatred.

Famous Fours include: Prince, Judy Garland, Bob Dylan, Edgar Allan Poe, Johnny Depp, James Dean

Type 5: The Thinker

A.K.A. The Investigator, The Innovator, The Observer, The Expert, The Specialist, The Mad Scientist

The primary need of a Five is the need to know.

The primary thought of a Five is "I can come up with a better way."

At their best, Fives are intellectual, analytical, perceptive, original, persistent, wise, and objective, but they can also be eccentric, phobic, arrogant or aloof, stingy, distant, critical, and stubborn. Fives possess incredible ingenuity, and are often creators or inventors—either of a "real" invention, or simply a better way of doing things. Fives must be careful not to be too put-offish or self-involved. The character "Doc" from *Back To The Future* is an exaggeration of the Type Five personality.

Fives grow by coming out of their intellectual mind to become more in touch with their emotional and especially their physical body. They need to discover a new sense of physicality and vitality. As they become more alive, they can begin to apply their intellectual creations in a more practical way.

Fives must be careful to avoid isolation, chronic physical neglect, declining hygiene, intellectual arrogance, eccentricity and loss of social interest, and hallucinations or distorted perceptions.

Famous Fives include: Vincent Van Gogh, Bill Gates, Charles Darwin, Tim Burton, Stephen King

Type 6: The Loyalist

A.K.A. The Guardian, The Doubter, The Troubleshooter, The True Believer, The Traditionalist

The primary need of a Six is security.

The primary thoughts of a Six are "I better do what's expected of me." and "Better safe than sorry."

At their best, Sixes are loyal, committed, likable, responsible, consistent, detail-oriented, practical, helpful, and warm, but they can also be nervous, insecure, masochistic, rigid, testy, judgmental, and controlling. Sixes are those people who will go down with the ship—hanging on to friendships and ideas to the bitter end. They tend to lack self-confidence, so they rely on others to feel secure. Sixes often become anxious when faced with making a decision or "going it alone." They are great "team players" and are much happier handling the finer details than being in charge.

Sixes grow by becoming more physically centered and grounded. They gain confidence and security simply by allowing themselves to fully feel the present moment. They also need to define security in more realistic and definite terms.

Sixes must be careful to avoid anxiety and panic attacks, feelings of inferiority, fear of loss, attachments to abusive relationships, hypervigilence, and suspicion or paranoia.

Famous Sixes include: Princess Diana, "George Costanza" (from Seinfeld), Rush Limbaugh, Tom Hanks, Malcolm X, Richard Nixon

Type 7: The Adventurer

A.K.A. The Enthusiast, The Generalist, The Multitasker, The Energizer, The Connoisseur

The primary need of a Seven is to have fun and contribute.

The primary thought of a Seven is "The grass is always greener..."

At their best, Sevens are enthusiastic, accomplished, uninhibited, fun-loving, spontaneous, imaginative, productive, curious and charming, but they can also be hyperactive, excessive, manic, impulsive, unfocused, rebellious, undisciplined, and self-destructive. Sevens are livers of life. They fully engage and love the finer things. Sevens come up with the most creative ideas, but can have tremendous difficulty following through or completing projects. Their zeal for life can often lead Sevens to self-destructive behaviors such as workaholism, overspending, and addictions.

Sevens grow by learning to slow down and quiet the rapid activity going on in their brains. Typical Sevens often have several thoughts occurring at once, which is why they can be scattered. Sevens can further advance by learning to focus on one project, task, or goal at a time—then following through to completion. Sevens must be careful to avoid disorganization and attempts to escape anxiety, addictions, impulsiveness, compulsive activities, being out of control, mania or depression, wild mood swings, panic attacks or paralyzing fears.

Famous Sevens include: Robin Williams, Steven Spielberg, Mozart, Jim Carrey, Jack Nicholson, JFK, Ben Franklin, Carol Burnett

Type 8: The Challenger

A.K.A. The Leader, The Protector, The Provider, The Maverick, The Entrepreneur

The primary need of an Eight is self-reliance.

The primary thought of an Eight is "I'm in charge. I know what to do."

At their best, Eights are powerful, decisive, direct, loyal, energetic, protective, and self-confident, but they can also be domineering, dictatorial, destructive, authoritative, bossy, controlling, and insensitive. The picture of the old-school CEO is an example of an eight. Eights can make incredible leaders, if they learn to be sensitive to the feelings of others. Some eights have a quieter demeanor, but still have the same strength and self-reliance.

Eights grow by learning to open their hearts to others. Children and animals often bring out the best in Eights, as this allows them to "let their guard down." It requires more courage for an Eight to share the warmth of his heart than to make major decisions. But this is the secret to an Eight's growth. Eights must be careful to avoid feelings of betrayal, social isolation, cold-heartedness, episodes of rage, violence, or physical destructiveness, plotting against "enemies", and antisocial or criminal behavior.

Famous Eights include: Martin Luther King, Jr., John Wayne, Sean Connery, Sigourney Weaver, Donald Trump, Barbara Walters

Type 9: The Peacemaker

A.K.A. The Healer, The Optimist, The Comforter, The Reconciler, The Diplomat

The primary need of a Nine is to keep the peace and avoid conflict.

The primary thought of a Nine is "Why can't we all just get along?"

At their best, Nines are easygoing, accepting, reassuring, pleasant, peaceful, patient, receptive, open-minded, and empathic, but they can also be passive, repressed, forgetful, "spaced out", apathetic, passive-aggressive, judgental, unassertive and lazy. Nines are the people who come in to put the pieces back together after a mess—at work, at home, within their circle of friends, or politically. In their desire to avoid conflict, they often fail to address important issues with others.

Nines grow by learning to recognize their own value, and by developing their own potential. Since they often go through life feeling "invisible", it is vital for a Nine to become more assertive and stand up for their own needs.

Nines must be careful to avoid denial of health, financial or personal problems, sense of inadequacy, dependency on others, emotional flatness, and feelings of disconnection.

Famous Nines include: Abraham Lincoln, Norman Rockwell, Walt Disney, Ronald Reagan, Whoopi Goldberg

There you have it! The nine Enneagram personality types. Did you discover your type? Did you immediately begin to think of certain people you know when you were reading each type? The Enneagram is not only fun but educational. It can also be an incredibly powerful way for you to blast through roadblocks in your life, learn how to get the most out of life based on your type, and learn to recognize the warning signs for your individual personality.

As this was a very brief introduction, I highly recommend further study. There are a number of excellent references, including the books mentioned at the beginning of this section.

Exercise

Use The Enneagram To Improve Your Life

Study your personality type to learn how to use your gifts to your best advantage while avoiding harmful patterns. Books on the Enneagram can help you grow and expand to a much deeper experience of life.

Learn What Makes Other Types Tick

Learn about the other eight types. This will help you better understand others and be able to better communicate "in their language".

Chapter 10

Stop Managing Your Time!

"And you run and you run, to catch up with the sun, but it's sinking.
And racing around to come up behind you again.
The sun is the same in a relative way, but you're older.
Shorter of breath, and one day closer to death."

The above words from Pink Floyd's blockbuster song *Time*, hit the nail on the head in a very creative way. One of our major cultural challenges, and one of the most common excuses for avoiding the life of our dreams, is the illusion of time. How often have you said, "I'd love to, but I just don't have the time." Or, "I'll do that someday when I have more time." Or "Let me see if I can squeeze that in."

But most of us *waste* far more time than we use. What? We all have far more time than we think, *at least far more time to do the things that we value most.* Before you run back to your stack of "time management" books and CD's, listen to what I have to say. Then you can make your own judgments.

We all want to achieve greater control over our lives. Most people believe that the best way to control our lives is to control or "manage" time. This myth has sold countless books and seminars. We even have a "Time Management" industry, as people spend millions on daily planners and fancy electronic schedulers.

Yes, we do need to organize or lives. And some jobs do require more strict adherence to schedules. But the experts have made a fatal flaw, and one that haunts millions every day. They believe the secret is *time* management. I believe this is incorrect. After all, time doesn't change, does it? You can't add hours to the day or days to the week. How can you manage something that you cannot change?

I believe the secret to getting the absolute most out of our lives is to manage ***our use*** of time. After all, it is ***what we do*** **in each moment** that determines the events of our lives, not time itself.

The Illusion of Time

There is really no such thing as time. The only "time" that truly exists is this moment. You can't change anything that has ever happened in the past, and you can't do anything in the future until *that* moment arrives. When we are busy rehashing the past or worrying about the future, we are wasting present moment after present moment!

How do you spend most of your present moments? Whisking the kids of to soccer practice... no music lessons... no the grocery store? Staying "busy" at work? Thinking about that deal you blew yesterday? Worrying about what will happen when the next car payment is due? All of these things paralyze us in "busyness" or in a state of fear. All of these things steal the present moment away from truly meaningful actions.

Most people attempt to control their time by having a "To Do" list. This should really be called a "Have To Do" list, because most of the things people write on their list are *things they really don't want to do, but "have to"*. Think about it. If you have a busy day at work, but are meeting friends at the ball game tonight, do you really have to write the following in your planner?

"Ball game—8:00. Leave house—7:00. Find parking—7:30"

Not unless you are completely insane! You'll know darn well when it's time to go. Why? **Because going to the game is something really important to you!** Most of us spend most of our time doing things we really don't want to do. In other words, **our lives are filled with activities that do not have anything to do with our purpose**. Because of this, we need a Have To Do list. We become slaves to our schedule. And in the end, ***time controls us***.

Do What Matters Most

Yes, there are things that we don't particularly want to do, but are necessary to our purpose. However, when you write or think about your daily list, do you start with the most *important* things or do you begin your list with the most *urgent* things?

Urgent and important are not the same thing. Urgent simply means that *if* you are going to do something, you'd better do it soon. Important means that it will have a significant impact on your life, your career, your finances, your family, etc.

Most people spend 90% of their day doing urgent things, and only 10% of their time doing important things. Is it any wonder why our lives are full of urgency, but little importance? Before you make any decision on how to spend your time, learn to determine what things in your life fit into each of the following four categories.

Important and Urgent:

These are activities that are both important and must be done soon. These should be your highest priority activities. Examples: Potential new client walks into office and says he is looking for a company to fill an order for several hundred thousand dollars. Your daughter has her piano recital in 2 hours. She has been practicing for months.

Important but Not Urgent:

These are things that may not need to be done right away, but are vital for your purpose. These activities may not be as high priority as the first category, but they must always be given priority over the urgent but not important activities. This is crucial to success and achievement! Examples: Planning a family vacation. Developing a marketing plan for your business. Personal development. Setting Goals. Exercising.

Urgent but Not Important:

This is the category that dominates most of our lives. We have been programmed to associate urgent with important, but this is not true. These tasks should be delegated to others, or not done at all. Examples: In the middle of creating your marketing plan, an advertising salesperson calls. She's only in town for one day, and really needs to talk to you about a "great deal" her company has going. You are playing catch with your son when the phone rings.

Not Important and Not Urgent:

These activities are pretty obvious—what most people immediately recognize as "wasting time".

In my Chiropractic practice, my receptionists know the number one rule: When it's patient time, **it's patient time!** This means that, short of a family emergency, I do not take phone calls, sales calls, or any other distraction while I'm caring for patients. Why? **Because taking the best care of my clients is the most important thing I can do to fulfill my purpose.** Likewise, when I'm working on a project (like this book), they know not to bother me with a question about a bill, or a Medicare submission, or anything else. So they take messages, set up appointments for sales calls, and set aside detail work I need to do—for a time when I am not doing something more important to my mission.

Are you beginning to understand why so many people are so stressed out by their mental or written "Have To Do" lists? They spend so much time doing less important things—or worse yet, *planning* how to get all of the less important things done—that they rarely get to the really juicy parts of their life!

Exercise

Are You Living Your Purpose?

Think about your purpose. Has most of your time today been spent fulfilling your life's mission? Or has your "To Do" list kept your focus and energies off purpose. Worse yet, are the things you are doing today actually preventing you from fulfilling your purpose?

If you don't remember your purpose word for word, that should tell you something. Go back to chapter 8 and review your purpose now.

Where Did The Time Go?

How many acres can a farmer plant in one day now, compared to 100 years ago (before the first tractor was built)? How much time (and effort) does it take to do a load of laundry in a Maytag washer and dryer compared to a hand washing machine, or a tub, or a river? How long does it take to get from New York to Los Angeles by plane, compared to horse-drawn wagon? How long would it take today for the Queen to find out Columbus had discovered the New World?

Technology has taken us a long way! Or has it? We seem to be busier and have less time every decade. So where did our time go? What happened to all the extra time we were supposed to have in a world filled with more and more conveniences?

Actually, we *do* have more time to create our lives than ever before. The problem is, we've filled up all that extra time, and then some, with relatively meaningless activities. The human mind craves stimulation. That's why children have such active imaginations, and why they explore. It is also what has driven the multitude of artists, and poets, and activists, and inventors throughout history. In the past, people had to humor themselves. They did this by writing, or painting, or spending quality time with family and friends.

Today, we are so stimulated by our environment (television, radio, video games, traffic, the office, gossip, and the evening news) that *we can't humor ourselves.* Spend 30 minutes quietly by yourself—no TV, no radio, no telephone, **nothing but your own thoughts—**and you'll quickly know what I mean! We are so used to being so stimulated so much of the time, that when we do have a moment of peace we find more clutter to fill it!

Now it's time to completely rethink the way you create your To Do list, in a way that will give **you**, not your schedule, control over your life.

The way to get the most out of your day, week, month, year, or *life* is to stop managing time and start managing your ***focus and priorities***. As we discussed previously, we get what we focus on most. A novice golfer hits great shots until she gets to the lake hole. Any tee shot she had made during the past six holes would have easily cleared the water. But not only does this next shot fail to make it over, it is a horrible shot that goes straight in. Racecar drivers are taught to focus on the track ahead, not the wall, during a spinout. When hockey legend Wayne Gretsky was asked what made him so successful on the ice, he said, "Other players focus on where the puck *is*. I focus on where the puck *is going*."

If you focus on all the "have tos" and "need tos", you will feel frustrated. When you start to focus on the "would love tos" and "wouldn't that be greats", your life will be filled with a renewed passion and vigor.

This is not a call to become irresponsible and do only the "fun" stuff. Not at all. Rather, it is an opportunity to create different *priorities*. It is a way to retrain your decisions when it comes to what to do with your time. Are you sick of the "rat race"? Have you had enough of feeling exhausted at the end of the day, even though half of your To Do list remains unchecked? Are you tired of feeling unfulfilled at the end of the day—even if you "got everything done"? If so, this next section provides a way to completely transform your life, to restore order, and to create the life you've been dreaming of (when you've had time to)!

Write Your Life's P.O.E.M.

Before we begin, there are two facts that we need to agree on.

Fact #1: It is impossible to do everything.

No one, not even superman, could possibly do *all* of the things he "should" "could" or "has to" do. It is physically impossible to do everything we want or other people ask us to do. This means that you need to *decide* what to do with your time. You will also need to decide what *not* to do with your time. There are moments when you need to say no.

Fact #2: Everyone can easily accomplish the most important things.

On the other hand, **everyone** (yourself included), can easily do *the most important things*. Think about it. If every day you picked two or three most important things, couldn't you get them done with time to spare?

It's simply a matter of choosing the most important, not the most urgent, activities. The POEM system will teach you how. POEM is a way to think and act in a way that is congruent with your life's mission and goals. It allows you to reprioritize your life so that the most important things always get done. And if the most important things always get done, your life will be immediately and forever transformed.

P is for **Presence**.

Presence means being here right now. Not just physically. Not just mentally. It means being physically, mentally, emotionally, and spiritually engaged in the Right Now. How often are you fully present? How often are you at work, but thinking about dinner? Or on a long overdue family vacation, but worried about what you're not getting done at work? Most auto accidents are caused because people are focused on something other than driving—not being fully present.

Being present is a natural state. We see it in children. It is why they can have a temper tantrum one moment and be laughing and giggling the next—as soon as their focus changes. It is why children have such a hard time putting their toys away—as soon as they're done with one, they're off to the next. Always present.

Over time, we allow the stresses, the pressures, the "busyness" of our lives to distract us from the present moment. So much, in fact, that very few adults are engaged in life anymore. Our lives are full of clutter and distractions. It's not a lack of *time* that causes stress, it's too much mental clutter, too many distractions, and too little clarity.

When we are distracted we are exceptionally inefficient. Even at times you don't realize, these distractions steal present moment after present moment. For example, your family is coming to town next week, and you have to get the house cleaned. So you create a great plan—start in the garage, then the master bedroom, followed by the living and dining rooms, the guest room, the kids' bedrooms and finally the kitchen. But the kids need someone to take them to practice. The phone rings. You decide to pick up that nice end table you've had your eye on. Someone at work calls in sick—so you go in on your day off.

Five days later... well, you've gotten started on the garage... and your guests are coming **tomorrow!** In desperation, you gather the troops. "Kid's, clean your bedrooms pronto!" "Honey, I need the garage cleaned!" You get right to work on the bedroom, the bathrooms, the living room, dining room guest room and kitchen. **Three hours later the entire house is spotless—something you hadn't accomplished in five days!**

This is the power of focus—of presence. Once you became fully present in the Now, all of your resources went to accomplish a single goal—to clean the house. And what happened? The house was clean in record time. What if your whole life was lived with this sense of presence? What if you played full out every moment?

There is an amazing description of the concept of presence in the book *The Power Of Now*, by Eckhart Tolle.

O is for **Outcome**.

What is the end result you really want from this present moment? Is it to eat, a vision for a new business, or quality time with your kids? Is it to gain knowledge and insight, so that your career can flourish? Or is it to simply rest and recharge? Every moment is designed for a unique outcome. Decide what it is that you really want.

E is for **Energy** and **Enthusiasm**.

If you remain fully engaged in the present moment, and focus on your desired outcome, it should be very easy to create the needed energy and enthusiasm. Get in the proper emotional state. Change your physical state (posture and breathing) to fit the goal at hand. You should have the same enthusiasm to change a flat tire as you do to open a Christmas gift. Changing a tire may not be pleasant, but the outcome—getting safely home—is just as important!

M stands for **Mission**.

"We're on a mission from God!" exclaimed John Belushi and Dan Akroyd in the classic movie *The Blues Brothers*. While their mission (saving the Catholic orphanage they grew up in) is different than yours, and although their approach was less than ideal, it was their passion for their mission that allowed them to beat all odds. What if you lived *your* life as though you were on a mission from God? You should, because you *are*!

What is that mission? Your mission is similar to your purpose. Actually, your mission is the specific ways in which you achieve your purpose. Instead of beginning each day with the much-despised To Do list, start only with the following two questions: **What is my life's mission and purpose? What can I do today to serve that mission and purpose?**

The answers to these questions are your *most important things*. Nothing else matters today, until the most important things get done. It makes no difference how much time you have spent on earth, or how much time you have left; **It's what you do Right Now that counts!**

Exercise

Live "On Purpose"

Write your purpose on something you can keep by your bedside or in your bathroom. *Every Morning* take a few minutes to become **Present**, decide what **Outcomes** you want today that fulfill your purpose, create tremendous **Energy and Enthusiasm** for the day ahead, and read your **Mission** out loud. Live "On Purpose" every day.

Procrastination—The Time Burglar

Procrastination robs us of our time. Because it is an issue of tim*ing*, most people falsely assume that procrastination is a failure to manage time properly. This couldn't be further from the truth.

Procrastination is caused by fear, and fear alone. Fear of rejection keeps us from returning that important call. Fear of failure keeps us from ever trying. Fear of success keeps us from taking the last step to complete a project. Fear of intimacy keeps us from saying "I Love You." Fear of inadequacy keeps us from saying "I'm sorry." Fear of confrontation keeps us from dealing with important issues. Fear of overwhelm keeps us from tackling that stack of paperwork. Fear of poverty keeps us from opening the bills or finishing our taxes on time.

These fears, and all the others, are really fear of pain. ***When we associate more pain with doing something than not doing it, we put it off. This is the root of procrastination.***

You may or may not realize that the act of procrastination actually creates more pain than "just doing it." Whenever you procrastinate, the delayed action or confrontation remains on your mind. All of the things you should be doing or should have done begin to build up (you can't fool "the man in the mirror"). This additional pain leads to further procrastination. Around and around you go. This state robs you of your present moments. Many if not most people spend the majority of their lives "wasting time" in this way. When your focus is stuck on the things you need to do but consider painful, you have less time to focus on what you really want.

Don't die with your music still in you.

A perfect example of procrastination is found in the shy boy at the school dance. He really, really wants to dance with a certain girl. So he sits there, planning his move. What will he say? What clever line can he use? How should he stand? What tone of voice should he use? But what if she says no? The more he wants to ask, the more his fear of rejection prevents him from taking action. So he waits and waits for just the right time (i.e. procrastinates). Finally, the music shuts down and everyone heads for the exits. He never did ask that special girl to dance.

If he had simply overcome his fear of rejection and immediately asked for a dance, one of two things would have happened. Either she would have said yes or she would have said no. Even if she said no, *at least he would have known*! But now he is tormented not only by the question of what she would have said, but also the misery of knowing that he didn't have the guts to ask.

All procrastination is some form of the "shy boy at the dance" syndrome. What's the solution to procrastination? It's *not* to do a better job of organizing your To Do list. Rather, it is about addressing your underlying fears.

Exercise

Stop Procrastinating, Start Living

First, determine what fears keep you from taking action. Are you afraid of rejection? Confrontation? Running out of money this month? Failure? Success...

List all of your action-stopping fears.

Then list all of the reasons that these fears are unrealistic, overblown, or unjustified.

Next, describe how procrastination actually *increases* the amount of pain you feel on a regular basis.

Finally, describe the positive impact taking action will have.

For example: Fear of rejection/ is unjustified because no one else can really reject me. I can only reject myself. Even if I feel rejected, the person is only rejecting my product or idea or company. They aren't rejecting me personally./

Not taking action will create more pain by not giving me a chance to close the deal. Sitting around wondering what the other person is thinking. Allowing me to create the worst-case scenario in my mind.

Taking action will make me feel powerful and in control. I will find out what the other person is thinking. I will know what my options are.

Procrastination-Causing Fear:

____

This fear is unrealistic, overblown, or unjustified because...

Not taking action will create more pain by...

Taking action will create pleasure or relieve pain by...

Procrastination-Causing Fear:

This fear is unrealistic, overblown, or unjustified because...

Not taking action will create more pain by...

Taking action will create pleasure or relieve pain by...

Procrastination-Causing Fear:

This fear is unrealistic, overblown, or unjustified because...

Not taking action will create more pain by...

Taking action will create pleasure or relieve pain by...

____
____
____
____
____
____

Procrastination-Causing Fear:

____

This fear is unrealistic, overblown, or unjustified because...

____
____
____
____
____
____

Not taking action will create more pain by...

____
____
____
____
____
____

Taking action will create pleasure or relieve pain by...

____
____
____
____
____
____

Chapter 11

Heaven On Earth—
Your Spiritual Connection

"Ask and it will be given to you; Seek and you will find; Knock and it will be opened to you."

Matthew 7:7

For centuries, "scientific" circles have considered it taboo to even discuss God or spirituality in the context of health. This is baffling. How can anyone have a legitimate discussion of the body's ability to grow, heal, function and adapt without involving the creative power that makes all of these things possible?

As was described in chapter two, 20th century medicine was dominated by *Mechanism*, the theory that the human body is a machine that can be explained through physics and chemistry alone. For spiritual, scientific and intellectual reasons, this theory has been entirely disproved.

As a result of this mechanistic viewpoint, Western culture has separated spirituality from science. The church is where you talk about God, but the laboratory is where "science" happens. Scientific advancements, including quantum physics and cutting-edge research, have brought God and science together. While we cannot specifically explain or define it, we now know scientifically that a vital force or intelligence exists.

Once you understand the theory of Vitalism, it is easy to talk about God (or however you define this life force) in the same realm as we talk about health. In fact, the two are *intimately and completely interwoven.*

So, let's shed the pretense that the mind, body and spirit are separate. Whether you are "religious" or not, it is vitally important to recognize the importance of your spirit and the source of that spirit. The very foundation of Chiropractic and Wellness is that place where body and spirit, science and God, meet.

Our Vitalistic Nature

Have you ever noticed your reaction whenever you come upon a newborn baby? No matter what's going on in people's lives, they drop everything to spend a few moments admiring, smiling, and making funny noises. Why is this? Because in a baby, we see the beautiful magnificence of God's love in its purest form. We are drawn like a magnet to the wonderful innocence of that creation—even when the baby cries, spits up, or worse!

If we choose, we can all create that very same magic in our own lives, every moment of every day. But we get caught up in our fragile egos and the hustle and bustle of life. So we choose *not* to admire the incredible creative force of the universe.

"If we could see the miracle of a single flower clearly, our whole life would change."

The Buddha

Exercise

Open Your Mind

Read a variety of religious/spiritual/inspirational books from a variety of authors. How do these books help to explain your own religious faith? How are they different. Do these books separate us on the basis of our religion, or do they point out our many similarities?

You don't have to fully agree with everything each author has to say, and you aren't required to make any kind of religious conversion. But let these ideas float around in your mind, then look at your own religion through your expanded eyes. If you are willing to do this, most people find a significantly deeper meaning and a closer connection within their own spirituality and religion.

What Life Requires

Human life requires but a few basic necessities:

Food

Water

Oxygen

Vital Life Energy, our spirit which flows through the body via the Nervous System

Which of these is most critical to life? Most people know that we can survive without food for a month or two, without water for a few days, and without oxygen for about 3-5 minutes. But did you know that life ceases to exist within **2 seconds** after the flow of nerve energy stops?

It is this innate creative force which allows us to express our full life potential. Unless it is disturbed. Whenever our connection to this vital creative force is compromised, our experience of life and health declines. This is why regular Chiropractic adjustments, which remove interference to the nervous system, have such profound and far-reaching benefits. It is also why it is so powerful to take the next step and strengthen your connection with your higher power, no matter how you define it.

Isn't Spirituality Just About Going To Church?

For many of us, our religion forms an integral part of our spiritual nature. However, being spiritual goes far beyond the act of practicing our religion. It involves looking more deeply into ourselves as well as looking for deeper meaning in our religious teachings. It involves shedding our own ego and realizing the greatness that lies within us—buried deep beneath our worldly image of ourselves. It involves being amazed by something as simple as a sunset. It involves being incredibly grateful for everything in our life—both good and not so good. It involves giving back to the universe—both in abundance and in actions. It involves recognizing that the entire human race is connected by our spirit, not separated by our differences. As Jesus answered the high priests, **the two most important commandments are to love God and to love your neighbor.**

Exercise

See Your Religious Experience In A New Light

From now on, when you celebrate your religion or go to church, think deeply about what the teachings are trying to say. How does this apply to *your* life? How does this apply to the world today? Is the meaning limited to what others have told you, or can you find additional lessons? Be willing to discuss different interpretations with your family. Do others see a somewhat different meaning? Rather than living in fear of your religion, or believing that there is only one way to interpret a particular lesson, expand your mind and open that conduit between yourself and God/source.

How Can You Strengthen Your Spiritual Connection?

By shedding your human ego. There are many tools, including prayer, meditation, congregational worship, reading, or simply observing the divine nature of everything! These practices have one common thread—they quiet our mind so we can observe what has always been right in front of us. The truth is that the harder you press, the more difficult your path will be. Simply allowing our awareness to take over allows our intuition to share its incredible wisdom.

There are many paths to spiritual enlightenment. You must find your own. So read, gain awareness, and listen to the insights that your intuition, or "God within" is telling you. Find different ways to discover your spiritual side. We recommend reading all of the books listed in the references and then some. Then revisit your religious teachings and note the deeper meaning they evoke.

"The power that made the body heals the body.
It happens no other way."

Chiropratic Principle

Exercise

Observe Other Practices

Many people have reported that some of their most amazing religious experiences have occurred when they have visited *other* denominations or religious services. By seeing how others practice their faith, we learn how closely tied the human race truly is. One of the most empowering experiences I have had was attending my cousin's Bar Mitzvah, where I learned a great deal about the Jewish faith and culture. Rather than weakening my own faith, it gave me an opportunity to grow and expand.

So, take a day to attend a religious service outside your own upbringing. Read books about other religions. Seek out people of other faiths and ask them what their faith means to them. You may be surprised to find that they are searching for the very same things as you!

Meditation And Prayer

Only a small percentage of people in Western cultures practice the art of meditation. This is unfortunate, as meditation is one of the most inspiring practices available. Perhaps the reason that so few people meditate is that they misunderstand what it is and what it does. What is your picture of meditation? Is it a monk surrounded by a circle of candles chanting for hours on end? This is what many people think—and also why so few learn how.

There are *many* ways and techniques to meditate. Chanting for hours is only one—reserved for a select few. Prayer is another, more popular version. Meditation is simply a way to calm the mind, clear out the clutter, and allow our intuition's creativity to flow or open the connection with our creator. Let's look at how Webster's Dictionary defines meditation:

> **Meditate—**to engage in contemplation or reflection. 1: to focus one's thoughts on : reflect on or ponder over. 2: to plan or project in the mind : INTEND, PURPOSE *syn*—see PONDER

Not so scary, is it? In fact, I'll bet you've "meditated" many times without even being aware of it. The art of meditation is to learn how to quietly allow your mind to flow, to ponder, to simply be aware, whenever you want! There are many good references, ranging from quick and simple relaxation to more advanced spiritual meditation. I'd like to share two techniques that I use. The first I developed for myself, and the second was developed by Dr. Dennis Perman.

Color Meditation:

Get into a comfortable chair in a quiet, dimly lit room with both feet on the floor, your shoulders relaxed, and your hands comfortably palms-up in your lap. You may want a partner to slowly read the instructions to you.

Close your eyes and envision the entire room, the entire world, engulfed in a single color—go from color to color until you find one that "sticks" or feels right.

Either quietly out loud or in your mind, repeat the name of the color over and over and over again. Do this until your mind begins to stay focused on that color only.

Next, shift the focus into your mind. The color should now engulf your mind as the room disappears from your consciousness. Focus on nothing at all except the color, and the name of the color.

After your attention has shifted inside, begin to *feel* your breath. Really feel the air flowing in through your nose, down through your throat, filling your lungs, and then exiting through your mouth. Picture the air as being the color you are focused on. Visualize this color coming in, filling your lungs, and exiting.

Now, picture this color flowing slowly through your body. First down your head and neck, across your shoulders, and down your arms and hands until it reaches every fingertip. Then through your chest and upper back down through your trunk, hips thighs, calves, and feet until it reaches every toe.

Finally, in the same order, allow that color to slowly leave—from your head, neck, shoulders, arms, and fingers, from your back, chest, trunk, hips, legs and toes—until there is nothing. Nothing except energy. Nothing except intelligence. Nothing except light.

Allow yourself to remain in this state until you are ready to return. Then allow the color to come back to your body, beginning again to feel your physical parts, then to your breath, then to your mind, and finally to the room.

Do not "fight" any thoughts or distractions that occur. Especially if this is a new process or you are stressed out, thoughts will likely pop into your mind. Simply be aware of them and let them float away. Whenever you feel distracted, come back to the color and remember to focus on the name of the color over and over again.

"White Noise" Technique:

The white noise technique can either be used as a regular meditative technique or a quick way to calm your mind in times of stress. Simply select the word or name that is currently on your mind and repeat it. For example, if you are angry at Joe for something he did and are emotionally fired up, simply repeat his name with your eyes closed over and over again until the strength of the emotional response calms down and the name Joe loses its power. If you have a lot of bills to pay, simply repeat the word bills until it loses its fearful effect on you. You can also simply pick a word to get a quick "clutter nap".*

There is no room for Wisdom in a cluttered mind.

Meditation is a time-honored practice which is designed to increase our awareness of what's real. It is a great way to remove the daily clutter from your mind, and to relax both physically and mentally. It allows the voice of God, or the universe, to come in. Recent studies have shown that expert meditators demonstrate real changes in brain activity—and even show changes in the way their brains are wired. This indicates that meditation actually creates a completely new state of awareness—a "sixth sense" if you will!

Exercise

Find a *minimum* of one thing you can do every single day to strengthen your connection with your source.

*I am grateful to Dr. Dennis Perman for sharing his White Noise technique with me and allowing me to share it with you.

Chapter 12

Living In Abundance

"God wants you to be rich."

Paul Zane Pilzer

More than perhaps any other factor, it is a *lack of financial freedom* that prevents most people from experiencing their dreams. This is caused by misunderstanding what money *is* and what money *means.* This leads to a frustrating and unfulfilling attempt to create a *lifestyle* rather than a *life.* Because of this, it would be impossible to create a complete Wellness Plan without a discussion of money and wealth.

Contrary to popular belief, wealth and abundance has very little to do with how much money you make. Being "rich" and being "wealthy" are not the same. Winning the lottery will not make you any wealthier than you are right now. On the other hand, using even a small windfall to create financial freedom, enrich your life, and contribute to the world will increase your wealth immensely.

Wealth and abundance are a *state of mind,* not a life condition! Like everything, it's an *inside-out* job. How you feel about money will determine your financial destiny far more than a promotion, lottery, or inheritance.

In this chapter, we will dispel the biblical misinterpretation that "money is the root of all evil." You will learn how to think abundantly and allow the universe to provide all the resources you desire. Finally, you will learn to use the *energy* of money to create your life just the way you want it. Why? Because you, like everyone else, deserve an abundant and fulfilling life.

Secrets of Wealth And Abundance

In their book, *Inspired Wealth,* Aileen Miga and Janice Hughes describe 12 principles of financial leadership*. We recommend that everyone, regardless of your age or current financial situation, invests in this book *before* doing anything else. This amazing books dispels the myth that financial success is simply an X's and O's strategy to figure out how to make more and more. It is about creating value by discovering who you are and using money to achieve your life's purpose. Since money is a form of energy, it naturally flows toward those who create increased *value.* The authors explain:

- Money is a symbol of appreciation, a gesture of good-will
- Taking care of your prosperity is paying attention to the energy reserves that you need to get work done, to fulfill your life's purpose or calling
- Money flows to those who give more in use value than they give in cash value. Money flows based on the exchange of energy. If we give more value to others the natural flow is to attract more energy to us, in the form of money, vitality or some other form of energy.

How often do you say to yourself, "I can't believe how expensive that is. There's no way I can afford it." How often have you complained about your phone bill? Or the price of gas? Do you look at your restaurant check and calculate the bare minimum you need to pay in gratuity? You may not realize it, but all of these things work against the universal laws of money, and are actually *preventing* you from gaining wealth!

Most of us are caught up in a world of instant gratification. Since we don't have a clear picture of what's most important to us, we tend to use money to keep us entertained, to "get us through the day", or to escape from the

* Aileen Miga, CFP and Janice Hughes, DC, LCP(hon), *Inspired Wealth: Financial Leadership for the 21st Century,* ©2004.

emptiness of our unfulfilled lives. The marketing and advertising industry knows this, so they dangle their carrots by trying to convince us that their product is exactly what we need to make our life "perfect".

But life is not about things. It's about fulfilling our most beautiful purpose. It's about relationships. It's about the experience. And at the end of the month, when we find we have barely enough to pay for all of those *distractions*, we realize that we are no closer to having the financial resources we need to have the *life* (not lifestyle) we truly desire.

"Money is the FUEL.
You are the VEHICLE.
Your goals are the ROAD.
Your vision is the DESTINATION."

Aileen Miga & Janice Hughes,
Inspired Wealth

I am not recommending that you live "on the cheap". In fact, hoarding money tells the universe that you are selfish, and the universe rewards you accordingly. I *do* recommend that you make congruent choices about what you use your money for and when. Use money for those things that truly enrich your life, rather than for diversions, distractions, and competing with the Jones's.

Exercise

Design Your Life

Review your purpose and biggest goals. Next, write a detailed list of all the tangible things that support the life you desire. What is your dream home like? When do you plan to retire? What do you plan to do after you retire? Do you have college educations to save for? Do you desire to become debt-free? What exotic places would you like to visit? What hobbies would enrich your life? What "toys" and luxuries would create fulfillment in your life? How much money would you like to donate? Where?

Next, you need to realistically figure out what it will cost financially to accomplish all of these goals. What income level will you need to achieve? How much wealth do you need to create? Remember to account for approximately 3% inflation for each year. If you are already at the necessary income level and are saving and investing at a rate that will produced the required amount of wealth, then it's simply a matter of planning and budgeting. If not, you have the opportunity to create income and wealth in the next exercise!

Total Wealth (Savings or Net Worth) Required:

1 year	$	5 years	$
10 years	$		
20 years	$	30 years	$

Annual Income Required:

1 year	$	5 years	$
10 years	$		
20 years	$	30 years	$

There are 3 basic steps to financial mastery. **The first step** is to simply learn how money works. There are universal laws which govern money and wealth—it is imperative that you follow these laws.

The second step is to start with the end in mind. Not just in terms of dollars and cents, facts and figures, but rather who you are at the end of the road. Take a minute to think about your eulogy. What would you most want people to say about you? "Johnny was a rich man, who had a big home, a fancy car, and a great investment portfolio," or, "Sally was a great friend, wife, and mother. Her love for others inspired everyone around her to do their very best. Her leadership and influence will last forever." Doing what you love most will inspire you to do your best, and will give you the energy and passion required to live the life of your dreams.

Most people do it backwards. They let *others* tell them what they're "good" at. They look for the *job* (Just Over Broke) that will pay them the most money the fastest. *Then* they try to convince themselves that they actually like this job or career choice! They blame their lack of happiness on the "wrong" position, the "wrong" company, and the "wrong" boss, rather than realizing that they are not doing what they truly love. So they change positions, bosses and companies, and finally change careers—in order to make more money. How insane is this?

"When you want what you want more than you fear what you want, you will receive it."

Alan Cohen

Instead, why don't we stop, figure out what it is that really fuels our passion, and then *figure out how we can provide enough value doing what we love to attract wealth into our lives.* Why don't we teach our children to pursue those things that inspire them, rather than raining on their parade, telling them to be "realistic", and convincing them to take on a "safe" career that they really don't love? This concept was best explained by an esteemed colleague and President of The Masters Circle, Bob Hoffman, D.C. He tells of a conversation he had with his college-bound daughter who was trying to figure out what career choices to make. He told her to "Find a career that matches your purpose and passion with your paycheck." What a profound statement, and one our children all need to hear.

"A musician must make music, an artist must paint, a poet must write, if he is to be ultimately at peace with himself. What a man can be, he must be."

Abraham Maslow

The third step is to create a game plan that will ensure that you have enough reserves of money and other resources to be able to paint your life with the exact strokes and the exact colors which will fulfill your highest calling. While all three steps will require searching and learning through books, coaches, etc., this third step requires that you find a coach who is knowledgeable on the subject of investment and wealth creation. We recommend a financial planner who takes a holistic approach, planning your *life* first. Visit www.inspiredwealth.com for further information.

Exercise

Increasing Your Value

What income level do you desire in order to live your life? $ ______

What is your current income? $ ______

In this exercise, simply get into an extremely relaxed and creative state. Let all of the day's mental clutter float away. You may even want to use one of the meditation techniques from the previous chapter. Now, let your *intuition* answer this one simple question: **How can I provide enough *value* to the world in order to receive the financial rewards necessary to live the life of my dreams?** Just let this question float around in your mind and patiently wait for the answer(s).

Remember, there are only a few ways to increase your value:

Increase the number of hours you work

Increase your efficiency

Work at a job or at tasks that are more valuable (increase your value-per-hour)

Leverage other people's time (own your own company or acquire a higher position)

Leverage other people's money (borrow money for real estate investing or your own business)

Creativity—create new products, services, procedures, or ideas that increase your value (intellectual property)

If, after completing this exercise, you find that you are working at a job or career that will not allow you to achieve your desired levels of income and wealth, ***this is a wake-up call!***

If this is the case, you must do one of two things. Either find a new career (which may involve going back to school or going into business for yourself) or create an additional income stream ("on-the-side" things like real estate investing, writing, a valuable hobby, etc.).

Some Ways That I Can Increase My Value

Other Opportunities To Provide Value And Create Wealth

A Real-Life Example: The Health Care Crisis

The recent economic turmoil surrounding the U.S. Healthcare System is a perfect example of improper understanding of money. Everyone wants to be healthier. The problem they encounter is that health and Wellness require a long-term outlook and investment. Rather than create and carry out a plan for lifelong Wellness, most people default to the quickest and cheapest (so they think) approach—drugs or surgeries to subdue their symptoms.

Most people don't realize the tremendous long-term cost of this approach. First, even if you have insurance, **we all pay for every test, every drug, and every surgery.** The reason health care has gotten so expensive is that we don't usually see how much we are actually spending. The second cost is the adverse effects of drugs and surgeries, which is now the leading cause of death in America. Finally, in trying to feel better right now, we miss the opportunity to address the real reasons we are sick, *which may have nothing to do with medicine or chemistry*. When we fail to act in the direction we want (health and Wellness), we end up getting what we don't want (sickness). In America, health has become a *liability* rather than an *asset.* It has also taken its toll financially, as we now spend more than 15 cents of every pre-tax dollar we earn on sickness care. In fact, *more than half of all personal bankruptcies in the U.S. are caused by medical bills!*

If we instead focused on supporting and improving our *health and Wellness,* we would vastly improve our lives, increase our contribution to the world, and save billions in health care costs. For the price of a bi-pass surgery, you could have *an entire lifetime* of regular Chiropractic care!

Universal Laws of Prosperity

In his bestselling book, *God Wants You To Be Rich,* economist and lay Rabbi Paul Zane Pilzer dispels the biblical misinterpretation that "Money is the root of all evil." He explains that God has created all of the resources we need, and has given us the unique capability to use our intelligence or *technology* to make seemingly limited resources endless. The bible actually states that the *lust* of money is the root of evil, meaning that money ill-gotten or ill-used is evil. Greed, or money for money's sake is evil. In other words, **the misunderstanding of the spiritual meaning of money and a lack of gratitude for the abundance God gave us is the root of all evil.**

Think of it this way. Would we be able to rebuild tens of thousands of homes destroyed by the recent tsunamis if there weren't people that had adequate reserves of money and time? How are your family relationships different between months when you are financially comfortable vs. months when you have trouble paying the bills? How would your children's lives be different if you were able to pay for their college education, rather than starting out tens-of-thousands in debt? Or if you were able to provide them start-up capital for the business of their dreams? How would your family's life be enriched if you were able to take a 2 week vacation anywhere in the world every year? How much more could you contribute to the world if you had $500,000 to donate to scientific research or Habitat For Humanity or another worthy cause? How would your community benefit if you were able to provide the money necessary to build a youth center? How would you feel if you worked only because *you love to,* not because you need the paycheck?

In her groundbreaking book, *The Dynamic Laws of Prosperity,* Catherine Ponder writes,

> "It is shockingly right instead of shockingly wrong for you to be prosperous. Obviously, you

> cannot be very happy if you are poor, and *you need not be poor. It is a sin.* Poverty is a form of hell caused by man's blindness to God's unlimited good for him. Poverty is a dirty, uncomfortable, degrading experience. Poverty is actually a form of disease and in acute phases, it seems to be a form of insanity.
>
> "Poverty fills prisons with thieves and murderers. It drives men and women to drink, prostitution, drug addiction, suicide. It drives potentially fine, talented, intelligent children to delinquency and crime. It makes people do things they otherwise wouldn't dream of doing... The sinful results of poverty know no bounds. That is one of the reasons why, as a minister, I have felt so strongly led to do whatever I can do to help people learn how to eradicate the sin of poverty from their lives."*

Get it? God wants you to enjoy the bounty She has placed before us. GOD WANTS YOU TO BE RICH! He also wants you to live with gratitude and use your abundance to contribute to the world. So *create great value* and willingly accept the rewards provided to you by an abundant universe. Then give back to the universe, with thanks, so that others may benefit from your bounty. Hoarding money, wasting money, and showing off money are all sins of lust. But creating wealth and lovingly distributing your wealth for the betterment of the world is the noblest cause you can undertake.

The Univeral Laws Of Tithing and Saving

Laws of money, that have held true for thousands of years, demonstrate the secret of wealth creation:

**Pay yourself 10% first. Give 10% back.
Live on the rest.**

*Catherine Ponder, *The Dynamic Laws of Prosperity,* Prentice-Hall, ©1962.

What this simple, yet powerful formula means is that you must pay yourself first! This tells the universe that you value yourself. You should save a minimum of 10% of your income every day, week, month and year. Put this money in a Wealth Account. The universal law of giving and receiving states that whatever you freely give to the universe comes back to you tenfold. This doesn't mean dropping a twenty in the offering plate on Sunday means that you will get a $200 lottery ticket on Monday. The universe isn't that direct. But it is an indisputable fact that the universe rewards generosity. Not just in money, but perhaps in health or a new friend. Just believe that this is true, and let the universe know that you are so grateful for what you have that you are willing to share—without strings attached.

"Give and ye shall receive."

Before you say, "I can't afford to save and tithe, I can't even pay my bills," remember that this type of thinking is exactly what prevents abundance from entering our lives. While no challenge is ever easy, the vast majority of people find that they do surprisingly well on 20% less. Tithing will renew your sense of contribution and you will begin to see all the ways that others contribute to *your* life. And as your Wealth Account grows, you will feel an increasing sense of comfort and security, allowing you to direct your inner resources to more productive activities than worrying about money.

Debt Reduction Formula

Most Americans have some form of debt. Sometimes, in the course of our lives, it is necessary to acquire debt in order to reach our goals. For example, most people require a loan to purchase a home or to start a new business. However, many of us find ourselves in a considerable amount of debt that saps considerable money energy. The average American family has about $8,000 in credit card debt and spends about $2,000 per year on credit card interest alone! We will show later how much wealth could be created by investing this money, rather than paying interest.

There are 2 secrets to debt reduction. The first is differentiating "bad" debt from "good" debt. Yes, there is such a thing as good debt. Good debt *makes* you money. This may sound illogical, so let me explain. Obtaining a mortgage to purchase a home costs you money in interest payments. However, homes generally *appreciate* at a higher rate than most mortgages. In addition, you can likely deduct this interest from your taxes. So, in the long run, *the money you spend on a home mortgage will create wealth, whereas the money you would spend in rent is simply lost.* Bad debt is debt that *costs* you money. This is especially true for credit card and consumer debt. But even a car loan is bad debt, as your vehicle will constantly *depreciate* in value.

Good Debt: Home Mortgage, Business Loan
Bad Debt: Automobile Loans, Credit Cards, Consumer Loans

The second secret to eliminating bad debt is a formula. It works like this:

Make all of your minimum payments each month. Determine a dollar figure of *extra* money that will be used for debt reduction each month. Budget in order to live on the rest. Now, use the *entire amount* of the money set aside for debt reduction to begin paying off the account with the *lowest balance.* Do this until the lowest balance loan is completely paid off. Then, with the original monthly amount set aside for debt reduction, *plus* the minimum payment you were making on the first loan, begin paying off the next lowest balance. Over time, the amount of extra money you have for debt reduction escalates dramatically, and you will be able to become debt free faster than you may think!

This is a proven formula for debt elimination. The secret is to stay disciplined every month!

Home Ownership

Owning a home is perhaps the most important thing you can do to create wealth. In most areas, you can pay roughly the same (often less) per month for a home mortgage than for rent. A home is one of the safest investments you can make. Historically, homes have typically appreciated in the 7–8% per year range. Today, home values in many areas are increasing much faster. You can write off interest payments on your primary residence. And there is no tax on the capital gains when you sell your primary residence (see your accountant and IRS guidelines).

The main reason people fail to buy a home is the down payment. However, most people can qualify for 90%, 95%, or even 100% or more financing. Many homes are now purchased with little or no down payment while keeping payments relatively low.

Lender	Loan Type	Balance	Minimum Monthly Payment
	Totals:		

Health Savings Accounts

As was discussed earlier in this chapter, the current system of insurance dependence has led to a stunning degree of financial mismanagement in Healthcare. More than 1 out of every 4 healthcare dollars currently goes to *administration* (paperwork). This is why most $2,500 deductible plans actually cost $3,000–$3,500 per year less than no-deductible plans. That's right! Even if you were to spend your entire deductible out-of-pocket, it is still usually cheaper than the equivalent no deductible plan!

In addition, the current system of low-deductible, low co-pay insurance and managed care has created a climate in which those who are *responsible* end up paying for those who are *irresponsible.* This creates a significant financial incentive to be *irresponsible.* In other words, if you are required to pay for things that improve your health, but get basically free care when you get sick, it causes a tendency to *wait until you get sick so your insurance will pay for it.* This is a major reason for our current healthcare crisis—doctors are no longer dictating what's appropriate, insurance companies are!

Help is on the way! It's called a **Health Savings Account** (also called Medical Savings Account, HSA, MSA). Health Savings Accounts will revolutionize healthcare, because they take away the financial incentive to be irresponsible. Passed by Congress in late '03, a majority of Fortune 500 companies already offer HSA's to employees. Private plans are also available from a number of insurance carriers.

A typical HSA works like this: Instead of having a low deductible insurance plan that can only be used for insurance company approved medical procedures, you have an account of typically $2,500–$5,000 which can be used for *any health or Wellness expense.* This means that **you**, the consumer, can choose exactly how you want to use **your** money! This can be for Chiropractic, supplements, massage, acupuncture, an M.D., D.O., etc. You can even choose your favorite providers—not whoever is on your insurance panel or your insurance company assigns to you. The amount of the savings account works as your deductible. When and if your spending goes above this level, your regular insurance kicks in.

So with an HSA, you are protected against major medical expenses, but can choose whatever healthcare fields and whoever you wish to see for your regular health and Wellness—no questions asked! HSA's are about the same cost as traditional managed care, and have significant tax benefits.

You should immediately discuss an HSA plan for your family with your employer, insurance agent, and financial planner or CPA.

Compounding Interest

It takes far less than you may think to create substantial wealth during your life. The table shows the amount of wealth created based upon a conservative 8% average rate of gain.*

Remember the fact that the average American family spends over $2,000 each year on credit card debt? If you simply kept your credit cards in check and invested the money you saved into your wealth account, *you would create an **extra** $300,000 over the course of your working life!*

*Dr. Larry Markson, Dr. Dennis Perman, and Dr. Bob Hoffman, *The Masters Guide For The 21st Century Chiropractor,* ©1999, 2000, 2001, The Masters Circle, Inc.

Yearly Savings	5 Years	10 Years	15 Years	30 Years
$2,500 ($50/wk)	$15,793	$39,260	$74,134	$325,000
$5,000 ($100/wk)	$31,586	$78,521	$148,267	$650,000
$12,500 ($240/wk)	$78,962	$196,303	$370,660	$1,600,000
$25,000 ($500/wk)	$157,930	$392,606	$471,335	$3,200,000

This table shows the power of compounding interest. Amounts are calculated based upon full re-investment of money and at a very conservative 8% annual rate of return.

Summary

Wealth and money is one of the most misunderstood concepts in today's society. The reality is this. No matter what your income level, you can *choose* to live in abundance or you can *choose* to live in poverty. By changing your concept of money, recognizing the energy and spiritual nature of it, and constantly striving to increase the value you create in your life, you can break out of the old depression-era mentality of poverty—and experience life in an entirely new way.

Exercise

Create Your Wealth Account

Create a Wealth Account (Mutual Funds, Savings, Money Market, etc.). Set aside a specific amount each month (ideally 10% or more of your earnings) to grow this account. Then never ever touch it!

Pay yourself 10% first (invest)
Give 10% back (tithe)
Live on the rest

Chapter 13

Raising A Healthy, Drug-Free Family

"Say No To Drugs!"

Our children are in trouble. You don't have to look far to see that our children are entering a very complicated world. You don't have to look closely to notice that our children are sick. Very sick. Diagnoses such as autism, SIDS, and ADHD did not exist prior to the 1940's. Childhood asthma, allergies, and diabetes, which were rare even 20 years ago, now occur in epidemic proportions.

What happened? What is causing this pediatric health crisis? Don't we live in the most medically advanced society in the world? Shouldn't our children be getting *healthier*, not *sicker*?

Parents blame teachers, teachers blame parents, the media blames society, and society blames the media. Certainly there are many reasons for the declining physical, emotional, and behavioral health of our children. Our modern lifestyle—poor eating habits, video games, and lack of exercise is one cause. Children also face increased stress—from violence at school and on TV, from increasingly complex family dynamics, and from pressure to succeed.

But doesn't much of the blame lie with those who have been entrusted with our children's health? After all, hasn't Medicine promised that they will keep our kids healthy? Don't they entice us with "Well-Baby" visits? Don't they brag about all of their advancements? Don't they condemn *anyone* who questions their authority, safety, and effectiveness—even people within their own profession?

If our children were getting healthier, the medical profession would be quick to claim victory. So why won't they take *any* responsibility for what has happened to our children? Quite the opposite has occurred. Just as our children have become sicker and sicker at the hands of dangerous medications, doctors prescribe more and more drugs, and pay less and less attention to the adverse effects. I have even heard of cases where children under the age of 3 have been prescribed antidepressants!

There is a large (and growing) body of scientific evidence which proves that severe, even deadly reactions to vaccines are much more prevalent than advertised. This body of evidence also points to a strong relationship between vaccines and many chronic neurologic and chronic conditions, including autism, asthma and allergies. Yet the medical profession and government agencies are using more force and stronger threats than ever. In order to coerce parents to get their children vaccinated, they threaten to keep their kids out of school. They threaten, slander, and ridicule other doctors, simply for sharing valid scientific research data with their patients. A local school nurse has even been lying to parents, saying that the exemption form (that she is required by law to provide) is "no longer available." And every year we vaccinate for more and more typically harmless childhood diseases.

In my state, chickenpox (yes chickenpox!) vaccination is being added to the list of "mandatory" vaccines. This is despite the fact that chickenpox is virtually harmless in children. And despite the fact that it is possible, if not likely, that this immunity will wear off in adulthood when the disease is dangerous, even deadly! This situation has already occurred with measles.

While nobody really knows the benefits of vaccines (because of a horrific lack of scientifically valid research), they *may* truly provide some benefit. However, the medical establishment has done little to answer this question and has purposely withheld information about significant risks. In other words, they have *prevented* parents from making informed decisions regarding their children's health.

For many decades antibiotics were, *as a rule,* prescribed for ear infections. Hundreds of millions of children were given antibiotics—*before sufficient research was completed.* Then a very large study was published more than a decade ago. It concluded that in most cases **antibiotics actually caused ear infections to last longer and return more frequently**. The treatment was doing more harm than good! And the serious problems associated with the overuse of antibiotics are now well documented.

But before this new research, guess what happened to professionals who disagreed with giving antibiotics for earaches. That's right! They were ridiculed, slandered in the media as "unscientific" and "dangerous", and often forced to the fringe of their profession! Despite this new research, and despite a CDC campaign to educate parents *not* to expect antibiotics for most ear infections, many parents still demand antibiotic prescriptions for ear infections!

It is likely that at some point in the future we will look at vaccination in the same light as antibiotics for earaches, bloodletting, lobotomy, and other failed (and often harmful) medical interventions. The multitude of doctors and scientists who are critical of vaccines will then be vindicated, much like the professionals who warned about the misuse of antibiotics have been today.

Chiropractors (along with medical doctors) vary widely in their *personal* opinions regarding the risks and benefits of vaccinations. The Chiropractic *profession in general* has held four consistent viewpoints regarding vaccines:

1) **More high-quality, unbiased research is needed.** We cannot continue to simply *assume* that vaccines are beneficial.

2) A large body of scientific evidence shows that the true risks of childhood vaccines are *many times greater* than is being presented to the public. **Parents must be told the truth, the whole truth, and nothing but the truth.** Failing to do so is providing medical treatment without informed consent.

3) Neither the chiropractor, nor the pediatrician, nor government agencies, nor the school nurse should dictate what a parent should or shouldn't, can or can't choose when it comes to their child's health. Most chiropractors believe that **parents should have the freedom to make informed choices regarding *their***

child's vaccinations and all other healthcare decisions. If a parent chooses to vaccinate their child, that's fine. But in a free country, it should be equally acceptable for them to choose *not* to vaccinate. If vaccines *do* work, how can non-vaccinated children pose any risk to vaccinated children? And if they *don't* work as advertised or are potentially dangerous, aren't parents entirely justified in choosing not to subject their children to a questionable medical procedure?

4) The decision whether or not to vaccinate should be based on the best available evidence—not rhetoric. This includes rhetoric from government agencies (who at their highest levels are controlled by people with close ties to—you guessed it—the vaccine industry).

Despite all the apparent doom and gloom, there *is* a way that you can ensure the healthiest, safest, and fullest life possible for your children. But you'll have to do it yourself. This chapter shows you how.

The Real War On Drugs

In a typical year in the United States, about 20,000 people die from illegal "street" drugs. Before being removed from the market, the prescription drug Vioxx® caused at least 30,000–40,000 known deaths—all by itself. Non-steroidal anti-inflammatories like ibuprofen cause more than 20,000 deaths each year due to intestinal bleeding. According to the most current research, at least 300,000 people die every year from medications alone. When deaths from surgeries, medical errors, malpractice, and other iatrogenic events are added, many medical researchers believe the total annual death toll from medical intervention to be nearly one million.

"What the [heck] is going on out there?!"

Vince Lombardi, Legendary Green Bay Packers Head Coach

In no way do I suggest that illicit drugs are ok or that our efforts in that area are unimportant. Nor am I suggesting that prescription drugs should never be used. But it seems a bit ironic to spend billions *fighting* the illegal drug trade while spending hundreds of billions *supporting* the pharmaceutical industry—especially when legal drugs cause roughly 15 times more deaths than illegal drugs. It has become obvious that *there is a complete lack of accountability within the pharmaco-medical industry.* Until someone else begins to take responsibility, you as a parent or grandparent will need to wage your own individual war on drugs.

Kids Aren't Dumb

Here is an example of a typical American child's experience with drugs.

Birth:

Johnny gets vaccinated for hepatitis B. Johnny will be injected with 45 different vaccines by 6 months, 64 doses by 18 months, and 74 by the age of six. Mom and Johnny are told that these shots will "make him healthy" (as if there is any reason to believe that he wasn't *born* perfectly healthy).

2 months:

Johnny gets fever after vaccination. Parents give him acetaminophen.

3 months:

Johnny has earache. Doctor prescribes antibiotics which are given for 1 week.

4 months:

Earache has returned. More antibiotics prescribed.

5 months:

Earache has returned. Stronger antibiotics prescribed.

9 months:

Johnny has a cough. Steroids and antibiotics prescribed.

12 months:

Earache has returned. Antibiotic prescribed.

15 months:

Johnny has runny nose. Mom gets "children's" version of adult cold medication.

Nose and sinuses remains plugged. Antibiotics prescribed.

2 years:

Mom complains frequently of headaches. Takes pills to "fix" the headaches. Johnny observes.

4 years:

Dad is grumpy. Mom explains that daddy is taking pills so he's less grumpy.

Possible strep throat. Antibiotics prescribed.

6 years:

Johnny begins having wheezing attacks. Goes to doctor. Diagnosed as asthma. Doctor has no idea what is causing it, but "lots of kids today have the same problem." Asks about family history in attempt to blame the asthma on genetics. Pills, steroids, and inhaler prescribed.

8 years:

Johnny is having difficulty learning and concentrating at school. Often fidgety and disruptive. Ritalin prescribed for ADHD. Johnny is told that he has a problem and the pills will help him sit quietly and learn better.

2 weeks later:

Johnny returns to psychiatrist. Mom says he hasn't been able to sleep much since starting on the Ritalin. Sleeping pills are prescribed. Johnny is told he has to take these at night to help him sleep.

6 months later:

Johnny is sitting still at school, but doesn't seem like himself. He has stopped playing his drums and painting pictures. He has lost weight and doesn't feel like eating much except Cheerios and peanut butter sandwiches. Doctor explains to mom and Johnny that these are common side effects, but that *not* taking the Ritalin "would surely be worse."

9 years:

Johnny's health and behavior problems have led to depression in mom. Johnny learns mom's new pills are to help "pick her up" and to "feel better".

12 years:

Johnny has severe relapse of asthma, and cannot participate in gym or sports. More powerful asthma drugs prescribed. Johnny has become very depressed because he can't play outside. Anti-depressants prescribed.

14 years:

Mom sits down with Johnny and explains how he should never ever take drugs because they are dangerous!

This is not an unusual story. In today's world, it is more typical than extraordinary. What do you think Johnny will do when his friends offer him pills that they promise will "pick him up", "mellow him out", or "make him feel better"? Sure his mother explained that street drugs are illegal and harmful. But his programming tells him that drugs are good for him, help him feel better, and help him fit in. Johnny has been programmed to use drugs to solve all of life's problems. How can we expect him to all of the sudden "just say no" to drugs?

Few, if any, medications prescribed to Johnny or his parents were even necessary! Most or all of the conditions treated with drugs could have been addressed *naturally,* by simply giving the body time to heal, using natural forms of health care, or by lifestyle or self-improvement techniques! Worse yet, it is likely that many of the health problems Johnny had were actually the *result* of overuse of medications. Do you think Johnny's opinion of drugs would have been different if he had been taught that his body and mind are perfectly capable of taking care of themselves nearly all the time?

Johnny, like so many of our children, is already a drug "user". For most of his life he has been taking one or more medications. Rather than learning how to develop naturally, his body has learned how to function *under the influence of chemicals*. If these medications were saving his life, that would be one thing. But this is rarely the case. We have sacrificed Johnny's *health* for his, his mother's, and his teachers' *comfort and convenience*!

Lead By Example

Your most important role is as a *role model*. Never forget that children idolize their parents and learn most of what they do by mimicking your actions. If you solve all of your physical and emotional problems by turning to drugs, this message is clearly imprinted on your children. At a young age, *it makes no difference whether the drugs are legal or illegal.* Children don't understand this concept.

One of the greatest lessons that Chiropractic children learn is that they have a tremendous built-in healing capacity. In order to help their body stay healthy, they learn to take care of themselves. This is very different than the lesson taught by Medicine, isn't it?

In a Chiropractic or Wellness-oriented household, children learn the value of eating right, exercising, and using medications only as a last resort. They learn that germs are just another part of the world, that 99.99% of germs are totally harmless, and that they have an immune system specially designed to fight of any of the "bad" germs. They learn to respect themselves, which makes it easier to respect others. They learn that a fever, while unpleasant, is their body's own attempt to fight off an infection. They learn that health is normal, sickness is abnormal. They learn that sometimes, some people need medications to help keep them going, but that drugs also cause harm.

By contrast, most households today are medically-oriented. Children are taught that people get sick because they have "bad" genes. They are taught that germs make us sick, and we are basically helpless against them, so we need antibiotics, antibacterial soaps, and vaccines to save us from germs. They are taught that being sick is normal, and being healthy is reserved for the "lucky". They are taught that drugs make us healthy and happy. They are taught that God made us "broken", and we need doctors and drugs to "fix" us.

The pharmaceutical industry understood this concept more than 50 years ago. If they could create the *illusion* that drugs are "good" and make us "healthy", and then convince parents, they would create a generation of highly dependant children. A generation programmed to reach for more and more medications. The pharmaceutical industry embarked on a long-term marketing campaign to create this exact cultural paradigm. They used fear of disease combined with huge pockets to enlist the medical profession and government agencies in this campaign. And guess what! Look around. They succeeded. Our culture is now addicted to medications. In fact, we now consume **dozens of times more medications than we did a just few decades ago!**

Unfortunately, what they promised and what they delivered ended up being completely different. What they *promised* was improved health and a better quality of life. The *results* are obvious by the statistics—Americans become sicker every year, and our world ranking for health has declined virtually every year. While some new treatments and medications have certainly saved lives, the vast majority have left a path of destruction in their wake. But every time more meds make us more sick, the drug industry is happy to dangle another carrot—in the form of *more drugs.*

I was just watching Extreme Makeover Home Edition (a great show that you should watch with your kids), when I was struck by two horribly slick drug ads.

The first ad was for Nexium®, a proton pump inhibitor (a drug that artificially shuts down the natural production of stomach acid). It stated that if you are over 60 and are taking pain medications for an extended period, "you may be at risk for stomach ulcers." Duh! Did they just figure this out? That's why they put the warnings on the label, and why you aren't supposed to take those drugs for an extended period! But never fear. Your doctor (the same person who is supposed to be looking out for *your* welfare) can help you continue to take your pain meds (going against label directions that warn against long-term use, of course) by *giving you another drug!!!*

The second ad was for an unnamed migraine medication praising the ability of their drug to "prevent" migraines. They had the gall to say that "Taking a medication after you get a migraine is treating the migraine, *but taking a drug every day is prevention.*" What?!? There's that catch-word, *prevention.* The Drug Industry clearly understands that people are now looking for *prevention* rather than *cure*, so they are now cleverly pretending like their drugs are preventive (i.e. keep you healthy). Remember—**every** medication has harmful adverse effects. The reason many drug ads don't name the drug is so they don't need to include the long list of harmful adverse effects.

And forget about trying to find or correct the *cause* of your pain or migraines. If you did that, you wouldn't need their drugs! It has become increasingly obvious that **the pharmaceutical industry has no interest in your health. Their only objective is shareholder profits. They just want you to consume lots of their product—no different than Coke or Microsoft or Chevrolet.**

So what can you do? First, walk the talk. Heal yourself first. Learn from your chiropractor and other sources the truth about how your body works. Learn how your Inner Wisdom is perfectly capable of taking care of you—as long as there is no interference. Take responsibility. Adopt a Wellness lifestyle. Do more outdoor activities with your children. Fix healthier meals for your family. Stay away from McDonalds. Forget the excuses. Our nine-year-old son's favorite place to eat out is Sweet Tomatoes (a large salad bar restaurant)! Above all, trust in your body's tremendous Innate healing capacity, and share this faith with your children.

What if you do have a medical condition that requires medication? First of all, determine if there is a natural approach that will reduce or eliminate the need for meds. There is a huge difference between taking insulin for diabetes and taking anti-depressants because you haven't learned how to handle the stresses in your life. Next, if you *do* truly need medications, use them privately. Don't make a big deal out of your condition or the fact that you need to take the medicine. Better yet, explain to your child that you have something going on that your body can't handle right now, but that you can't wait to get off the medicine.

Your child will model your approach to health—whatever that approach is. It's also important to teach your children the truth about medicine—that once in a while the body needs some assistance, but that all drugs have harmful side-effects. Your child will also learn from your lifestyle. If you smoke, it's more likely they will smoke. If you eat right and exercise, it's more likely that they will eat right and exercise. If you solve your problems with medications, so will they. If you yell and scream, they will yell and scream. If you let them know how much you love them, they will let you know how much they love you. It is important to remember that these habits, good or bad, last into adulthood. In other words, children from health-oriented families have healthier lifestyles when they grow up.

I love the saying, "Your actions speak so loudly, I can't hear what you are saying!" Lead by example. Take your role as a role model seriously.

Utilize Natural Health Care First

Just because your child gets the sniffles doesn't mean they are sick. Your child's immune system is learning and developing. It needs some exercise in order to get strong. Don't become alarmed at the first sign of a cold or earache. The last thing you want to do is interfere with the normal natural development of the immune system. Studies have shown, for example, that children who are exposed to more infections when young (at day care or having older siblings who go to school) have a significantly lower risk for childhood asthma and allergies later on. This being said, use common sense when there might be a more serious condition.

If you haven't already done so, you should have all of your children screened for subluxations, regardless of the presence or absence of symptoms. Your chiropractor can catch early signs of scoliosis or other spinal problems, and can determine whether or not your child's nervous system is working properly. Certainly, any child who has persistent or multiple health issues should be checked at once. Remember, **the choice is always yours whether or not to pursue health care of any kind for your child**. But get informed before making that decision.

Fever

One of the most absurd and unscientific dogmas spread by the mechanistic medical establishment is that fevers are bad. Many parents are advised to treat even low-grade (100°–102°) fevers with medicine designed to bring the fever down. This idea is so engrained that you are probably wondering what I am talking about.

Here's the lowdown on fever that your M.D. never told you. *The infection doesn't cause the fever.* **Fever is a natural defense mechanism designed to help the immune system eliminate an invading organism.** That's right! The body creates the fever *on purpose.* Far from being a sickness, a fever indicates that your child's innate defense system is working to restore her health, just the way nature intended. While it may make you feel "like you're doing something to help", do you really think short-circuiting a natural defense mechanism is going to help your child get healthier quicker?

I'm sure you've had the experience of having a fever (and feeling miserable), then the fever "breaks" and you almost instantly feel much better. This is your Innate Intelligence working at its best.

This doesn't mean that you should ignore a fever. A low-grade fever (up to 102°) means that your child needs rest in order to recover. Also, make sure they get plenty of fluids (unsweetened and no caffeine, of course). Also your child should consume mainly fruits and vegetables, or natural juices, as these contain natural substances that support the immune system. No sugar, as sugar provides an ideal meal for the offending germs. Also, temporarily avoid dairy, especially if there is a lot of mucous involved.

A mid-grade fever (102°–104°) means that there is a significant battle going on. This is ok, but you should closely monitor changes in temperature. When the fever exceeds 104°, it's time to begin getting a little concerned. However, recommendations have generally been skewed on the side of over-caution. The younger the child, the higher a fever can reach before becoming dangerous. In adults, 104°–105° begins the risk area. However, in young children it is rare to see any damage before 106°–107°. While there are very real risks with high fevers, and these are well publicized, the risks involved with giving medications may actually be much greater.

This being said, I would never recommend taking *any* chance, no matter how slight, with your child's health. So if your child's temp reaches 104°–105°, it's time to consult with your M.D. But use natural approaches first. Once the fever approaches 104°, try cool, damp washcloths or sponge-baths. Or, use some rubbing alcohol to naturally cool the body. And of course, closely monitor your child's temperature.

With a fever, as with most other symptoms, it is best to first monitor and give the body time to heal, second use non-invasive natural approaches, and finally use more invasive treatments as a last resort. If you follow this recipe, you will give your child's natural defenses an opportunity to work, while reducing the likelihood of harmful drug effects. And by using common sense, you will know when to take further action. By understanding when to leave well enough alone, and knowing when something more aggressive needs to be done, your child will have the best opportunity to heal—with the least amount of risk.

Teach Self-Respect

After our cultural addiction to medications, the leading cause of drug abuse is a lack of self-respect. Children (and adults) who have a healthy respect for themselves rarely turn to drugs.

Your child's self-esteem can be measured in three categories: Respect for their body, respect for their mind, and respect for their spiritual being. Body-respect can be summed up in the following statement: What you put in your body and do to your body will either heal it or harm it. The Wellness model teaches children that we are responsible for the things we consume and the things we do or don't do. God only gave us one body—it is our duty to maintain it as well as possible. If we don't, we have no right to complain about getting sick or feeling rotten.

Mind-respect relates to how your child feels about herself as a person. Parents, teachers, and peers tend to nit-pick about perceived "negatives". Whether you know it or not, this wears on kids tremendously. This is the reason for peer pressure. It is imperative that you teach your child that they are perfect just the way they are. Instead of telling kids they are learning disabled, lazy, or underachievers (all of which simply mean "bad" to a child), we should focus on the talents and skills that they *do* posses.

Some children are book-smart. Others are talented musically. Still others are athletically gifted. Some are very creative, while others are socially advanced. **Not everyone is destined to be an electrical engineer or a research scientist.** The quicker we learn this, the sooner we can appreciate each of the wonderful gifts our children have to offer. If learning is so important, why have you, the role model, stopped? Children should be encouraged to do their best at school, but don't berate your child if they lack the ability or desire to get top grades.

Spirit-respect is something adults tend to reserve for themselves. We falsely assume that children are too young to understand. So we drag them to church, kicking and screaming, without ever explaining *why*. Worse yet, many religious organizations teach our children that they are "bad", that God is "mean", and that they have to somehow "impress" God to get to heaven.

Do you see a pattern here? We all want our children to be happy, respectful, and grateful. But nearly every lesson our children learn is that they are "bad", "broken", or "evil". Is it any wonder kids are confused?

Whether or not you attend an organized religion with your child, it is imperative that they learn that God loves them and that God put them on earth to be happy and successful and to make the world a better place. Teach them that God gave each of us different talents in different areas, and our job is to do our very best with those talents. Teach them that the world is a loving place. And for crying out loud, **turn off the evening news and the "bang bang—you're dead" movies and video games!** Is this really the world you want your child to experience?

Raising A Healthy, Drug-Free Family—The Wellness Way

If you want a different result, you will need a different approach. Thankfully, there is already an established system of health care that has helped millions of children grow up with healthy bodies, healthy minds, and healthy attitudes. This is the same Wellness-based approach we have described throughout this book.

This chapter first exposed many of the reasons that our children fail to achieve health and happiness—and why they turn to drugs. Then, basic concepts were introduced to help you help your children make the most of their lives. Now, let's wrap things up by providing a recipe for better health.

Most of the information you will need to raise a healthy, drug-free family is contained in the pages of this book. The same principles apply to your children as apply to you. So make your children a part of a Family Wellness Plan. Let them learn as you learn (at their own pace, of course). Specific guidelines for your children are as follows:

Make careful, informed choices about *any* course of health care for your child. You are the parent, and ultimately you have both the right and responsibility to determine what to do (or not do) with your child's health.

Teach *Wellness* principles, not *Sickness* principles in your home. Limit talk about symptoms and medications. Use medications *appropriately,* meaning in emergencies or when nothing else works. Teach your child to trust in their own ability to heal, and the vital importance of taking care of themselves. Teach them that symptoms are unpleasant, but sometimes necessary for their body to heal.

Eat a healthy diet. This means *everyone*. Once they reach the age when they can eat solid foods, *all* children should eat the same healthy foods as the rest of the family.

Never fix a separate meal or a separate dish for one or more children. This is a recipe for disaster, as they will learn to *expect* to be able to eat whatever they want. No child has *ever* starved with food in front of them. If your child refuses to eat, simply say "OK," put the plate in the refrigerator, and let them know that when they are ready, they can eat. Then stand firm. There is to be no negotiating for alternate foods. What's the worst that can happen? Your child will go to bed hungry for a night or two. This won't hurt them a bit. And I guarantee that within a short time your child will eat what's on their plate! On the other hand, don't berate them or "force" them to eat something they don't want. Simply make it clear that they eat what's there or nothing. Then let *them* make that choice. Finally, allow your kids to participate in meal planning—it gives them the control they are looking for. "Would you like green beans or salad for our vegetable tonight?"

Keep the junk food out of the house. Go through your cupboards and refrigerator right now, and look at all the harmful foods you find. Then throw out the junk. Children do *not* have an extra food group called "chips", "cupcakes" or "popsicles". The best way to keep yourself, and your kids, from eating junk food is to keep it out of the house!

Promote an active lifestyle. Plan plenty of outdoor activities with your kids. *Reward*, don't punish active behavior. We live in a culture where children are expected to act like adults. Why? American adults are overweight, exhausted and depressed. Ever wonder why? Allow your kids plenty of play time—this is just as important to their development as reading or schoolwork. Limit TV and video game time. There is nothing wrong with a family sitting together and watching a healthy TV show (again, our favorite is Extreme Makeover: Home Edition because of the heartwarming lessons it teaches). The problem occurs when sitting activities take over for real exercise. Invest in products for your kids to use—balls, drums, trampolines, bikes, etc., rather than products that contribute to a sedentary lifestyle. Finally, there *are* certain times when sitting still is a priority (dinner, church, class). At other times, allow your child to move around—even if it drives *you* crazy. Movement is normal, natural, and healthy for kids!

Provide quality family time. This time is separate from outdoor activities. Dedicate an adequate amount of time each week to just being a family—talking, working out differences, laughing, setting goals, making plans, and teaching your kids the valuable lessons of life.

Paint a beautiful picture of the world. If your child believes that the world is a wonderful place, filled with mostly wonderful people, created by a God that loves them, they are far more likely to treat themselves and others with love, compassion, and respect. They will also be happier.

Involve your children in self-empowering activities. Obviously, this is age appropriate. But think about this: How might *your* life be different today if someone had shared these lessons with you when you were young? Empower your children to achieve anything in their wildest dreams. Our nine-year-old does affirmations, has written goals, has a success journal, and listens to CD's on a regular basis! We even have discussions (with him providing excellent input) about such things as the philosophy of *The Matrix*! One point, however. Children typically have much shorter attention spans than adults (this is a normal part of their development, not a "disease"). Therefore, keep these sessions short enough to keep your child's interest (no more than 15–30 minutes at a time). What are the best activities for kids?

<u>0–5 years:</u> Passive (listening) activities

Classical music

Affirmation CD's such as *"I'm a lovable me"*, *"Baby Einstein"* videos

Positive parent talk ("I love you", "I'm so proud of you", "You are such a good girl")

Begin simple affirmations like "I love myself", "I am a princess", and "I am a good boy"

<u>5–10 years:</u> Begin basic active involvement

Introduce concepts of goals (at this time, most goals will be "When I grow up I'm going to be a football player… no, an astronaut… no, an explorer") Don't rain on their party or try to get them to be "practical". All accomplishments start with a dream, then a goal, then action.

Help your child create their own personal affirmations that they say every day

Start your child thinking about *why* people do the things they do—"why do you think you got so angry?" "Isn't it wonderful that all those people helped build a nice new home for that family!"

Teach your child to daydream. Yes! Contrary to popular belief, daydreaming is not a waste of time. It's how all the possibilities in your child's life begin to unfold in his mind. The best nation in the world is... *Imagi*nation!*

11–17 years: Prepare for life

This age provides a transition from the unreal (childhood dreams) to the real (goals and plans for life).

Help your child discover their *passion*. Passion is their path to heaven. Help your child experiment to find what it is that they love doing.

Help your child redefine their goals in more concrete terms—based on their passion.

Teach your child about money—abundance, investing, wealth creation, the high cost of credit cards, etc.

Have your child expand into more complex areas of personal development.

There you have it! The recipe for a healthy, drug-free family. Does following this approach mean that their won't be challenges? Of course not. Children have a fierce desire to discover who they are. They want to discover for themselves what they can and can't, should and shouldn't do. Other adults, who don't understand Wellness the way you now do, may not understand. Your parents, your doctor, your friends may even get angry with you and your choices. But if you handle these challenges with determination and raise your children with love, you will give them the best opportunity for the kind of life their peers can only dream of.

*Thanks to Dr. Bob Hoffman for this pearl of wisdom.

PART 3

A NEW MODEL OF WORLDWIDE WELLNESS

Chapter 14

The Wellness Formula

"Every Day You Are Faced With Two Choices:
Live Your Life Or Begin To Die."

Brad Burke, D.C.

This book was designed to create a new awareness for you, the reader. An awareness of all that is possible. How you use the information is up to you.

So what's the secret to a life of Wellness? While every human being is unique and will utilize different tools during different phases of their life, this formula will provide the best opportunity for a maximum experience of life.

It really boils down to your choices, decisions, and level of commitment. Living a truly outstanding life is not as difficult as it seems. It is truly rewarding and exhilarating. But you can't run the race if you refuse to leave the starting gate!

The Wellness Formula

1) **Keep your spine and nervous system in tune.** This is the most important aspect of your health and life experience. Regular Chiropractic adjustments allow full expression of life.

2) **Get an attitude adjustment.** You cannot control what life gives you. But how you respond to challenges is a choice that you will make every day of your life. You have the choice between a life of happiness, gratitude, fulfillment, kindness and joy or a life filled with fear, grief, misery, envy, hatred, and regret—*regardless of your life conditions.*

3) **Get active and exercise.** Motion is life and life is motion. The ultimate lack of motion is rigor mortise!

4) **Eat foods that nourish you. Avoid foods that slowly kill you.** Good nutrition is key to a long and healthy life.

5) **Live with an attitude of gratitude.** When you are grateful for your life and everything it brings, you will have a renewed sense of joy and happiness.

6) **Manage your finances wisely.** Think abundantly, and use your resources to live your purpose.

7) **Work on yourself every day.** Perhaps the most important, and certainly the least utilized tool for a successful and joyful life.

8) **Get in touch with your spiritual side.** Connect with source on a daily basis.

9) **Avoid medications and other risky medical interventions.** Make appropriate decisions regarding your health care. While there may be times when medications are truly necessary, never forget that *every drug introduced into your body causes harm.*

10) **Live "On Purpose".** Clearly define your mission in life and live your purpose every day.

Epilogue

The Chiropractic Vision: Creating Wellness For Our Planet

"Never doubt that a small group of thoughtful, committed citizens can change the world; indeed, it's the only thing that ever has."

Margaret Mead

For the past 110 years, Chiropractic has shared a vision of Planetary Wellness—A healthier, kinder, more grateful and responsible human race. While the struggle has at times seemed insurmountable, the human race is becoming increasingly ready for a major paradigm shift. Nowhere is this more apparent than in the current transition from sickness care to Wellness.

In the early part of the 20th Century, due to the power of the American Medical Association, many chiropractors were jailed, simply for practicing Chiropractic. During the 20th Century, the public perception of Chiropractic changed from a "religion", to "unscientific", to "almost doctors", to "back pain and headache doctors".

I believe that the world is now ready to see Chiropractic for what it truly is: an Art, Science, and Philosophy that *understands* the vitalistic nature of life, *honors* and *trusts* the God-given wisdom possessed by every cell of our body, *maximizes* life and health by restoring nervous system integrity, and *empowers* us to take control of our own health through self-responsibility and informed choices.

Leaders within the Chiropractic profession share a vision that every child born into this world may have the opportunity to live a full, healthy, and successful life through the power of Chiropractic. We envision a day where the glow of Wellness destroys the darkness of sickness, where love replaces fear, where unity replaces separateness, and where peace replaces war. The Chiropractic lifestyle embraces all things that promote Wellness, wholeness and togetherness.

That day will come. How quickly it comes depends on *you*. Will you strive to become everything you can be? Or will you choose to remain trapped in a world of mediocrity? Will you choose to live in love, joy, abundance, and gratitude? Or will you choose to live in fear, frustration, scarcity, and envy? Will you share your experience and new-found wisdom with everyone you know? Or will you keep the Chiropractic Wellness Lifestyle a secret? The choice is yours, and yours alone.

Change Yourself and Your Family Changes

Change Your Family and Your Neighborhood Changes

Change Your Neighborhood and Your Community Changes

Change Your Community and Your State Changes

Change Your State and Your Nation Changes

Change Your Nation and The World Changes

Change The World and The Universe Rejoices

So

Change Yourself and Make God Smile!

References

Literally thousands of books have been written on the subject of human development. My all time favorite is ***Awaken The Giant Within*** by Anthony Robbins. This is a comprehensive, life-changing book that I recommend for everyone.

While every book on this list is excellent, I have noted a few that are my personal favorites.

◊ = Most Highly Recommended

• = Short and Easy To Read

Personal Empowerment

Awaken The Giant Within—Anthony Robbins ◊

Chicken Soup Series—Jack Canfield and Mark Victor Hanson

Clearing The Clutter For Good Feng Shui—Mary Lambert

Don't Sweat The Small Stuff—Richard Carlson •

Failing Forward: Turning Mistakes Into Stepping Stones For Success—John Maxwell

How To Win Friends And Influence People—Dale Carnegie

Notes From A Friend—Anthony Robbins •

The Breakthrough Experience: A Revolutionary New Approach To Personal Transformation—Dr. John Dimartini

The Highest Goal: The Secret That Sustains You In Every

Moment—Michael Ray & Jim Collins

The Magic Of Thinking Big—David Schwartz

The Six Pillars Of Self-Esteem—Nathaniel Branden

The 7 Habits Of Highly Effective People—Stephen Covey ◊

The Success Book—John Randolph Price

The Wisdom Of The Enneagram—Riso & Hudson ◊

Wonderful Ways To Be A Family—Judy Ford •

Spiritual / Inspirational

Awaken The Buddha Within: Tibetan Wisdom For The Western World—Surya Das

Conversations With God (Books 1, 2, and 3)—Neale Donald Walsch

Count Your Blessings—Dr. John Dimartini

Ethics For The New Millennium—The Dalai Lama

Everyday Enlightenment: The 12 Gateways To Personal Growth—Dan Millman

Journey To Center: Lessons In Unifying Body, Mind, and Spirit—Thomas Crum

Manifest Your Destiny: The 9 Spiritual Principles For Getting Everything You Want—Wayne Dyer

Real Magic—Wayne Dyer

Spiritual Literacy: Reading The Sacred In Everyday Life—Brussat

The Bible (or your religious guide) ◊

The Four Agreements—don Miguel Ruiz ◊•

The Monk Who Sold His Ferrari—Robin Sharma

The Power Of Now: A Guide To Spiritual Enlightenment—Eckhart Tolle ◊

The Seven Spiritual Laws Of Success—Deepak Chopra ◊

Wealth and Abundance

God Wants You To Be Rich—Paul Zane Pilzer

Inspired Wealth—Aileen Miga & Janice Huges ◊•

Rich Dad, Poor Dad: What The Rich Teach Their Kids About Money That The Poor And Middle Class Do Not—Robert Kiyosaki ◊

The Abundance Book—John Randolph Price

The Automatic Millionaire—David Bach

The Dynamic Laws of Prosperity—Catherine Ponder

The Millionaire Next Door—Thomas Stanley & William Danko

The Richest Man In Babylon—George Clasen ◊•

Think & Grow Rich—Napolean Hill ◊

Unlimited Wealth—Paul Zane Pilzer

Health & Wellness

There are numerous excellent books available about natural healthcare options such as massage, acupuncture, herbal remedies, etc. These are available at any major bookstore. There are unlimited references in the area of exercise and active lifestyle. I recommend that you first determine your areas of interest, then go to the bookstore and thumb through books on the subject until you find a book you like. Sometimes people become interested in a particular activity because they read a good book or article about it.

A Clear Path To Healing—Weinberg

A Shot In The Dark— Barbara Loe Fischer

Body For Life—Bill Phillips

Chiropractic First—Dr. Terry Rondberg ◊

Health and Nutrition Secrets That Can Save Your Life—Russell Blaylock ◊

On The Take: How Medicine's Complicity With Big Business Can Endanger Your Health—Jerome Kassirer, M.D. ◊

Sleep Disorders and Sleep Relaxation CD—Brenner and Goldberg

The Biology Of Belief—Dr. Bruce Lipton ◊

The Master's Guide For The 21st Century Chiropractor-The Masters Circle, Inc.

Some types of books you may consider are:

Books about Yoga

Books about Tai Chi

Books about Sports (golf, tennis, etc.)

Books about Martial Arts

Books about Hiking our National Parks

State Parks Department handouts and booklets on local hiking trails, etc.

Travel Catalogs

Books about inspirational personal stories

Books about using an exercise ball

Index

F

G

H

I

M

N

O

P

S

T

V

W

Printed in the United States
76160LV00002B/111